Discourses of Disruption in Asia

DISCOURSES OF DISRUPTION IN ASIA

Creating and Contesting Meaning in the Time of COVID-19

Edited by

Ikuko Nakane

Claire Maree

Michael C. Ewing

LEIDEN UNIVERSITY PRESS

Cover design: Andre Klijsen
Cover illustration: iStock.com/mammoth

ISBN 978 90 8728 423 7
e-ISBN 978 94 0060 466 7 (e-PDF)
https://doi.org//10.24415/9789087284237
NUR 740

Printed and bound by CPI Group (UK) Ltd, Croydon, CR0 4YY

Table of Contents

Preface and Acknowledgements

This volume emerges from collaborative research during the global pandemic by members of the Language Dynamics in the Asia-Pacific Research Cluster, Asia Institute, University of Melbourne. As borders closed and movement was restricted, even from our relatively privileged positions and being able to work from home during lockdowns, we struggled like many of our colleagues to find a balance between the expectations of teaching and research. Our monthly meetings were a source of support and collegiality that sustained us during difficult times, and we acknowledge the support of the Language Dynamics in the Asia-Pacific Research Cluster at the University of Melbourne. Thanks in particular go to Patrick Murphy and Tarek Makhlouf, who managed the administrative aspects of these gatherings while juggling their own PhD research during a pandemic. We thank our research assistant Tim Johannessen. We also thank the Asia Institute for its ongoing support of the research cluster, and this publication. We thank the Faculty of Arts for publication support.

Sections of some chapters were presented at "Quarantine, masks and dis/ease: social discourses of COVID-19 in Japan and Korea" on November 5, 2020. Many thanks to our colleague Melissa Conley Tyler (Research Fellow, Asia Institute) who chaired this session, and to Cathy Harper, Editor in Chief of the *Melbourne Asia Review*.

A note about the rendering of diverse languages across the chapters: as language specialists working in languages from the Asia region and writing in English, we have attempted to make the text as accessible as possible. Within the chapters, citations and examples are given in the source language, followed by a transliteration and translation. All translations are by the author of the chapter, unless otherwise stated.

Edited books are a product of collaboration and collegiality. We thank our contributors for their generosity in sharing their time and expertise. Without your support and assistance none of this would have been possible. We thank Ben Morgan for his excellent assistance in editing. We thank the anonymous reviewers whose comments we have taken on board as much as we can. We acknowledge and thank our editors at Leiden University Press: Romy Uijen, S.M. Gieling, Lisa van Vliet. Your patience in fielding questions and offering advice is very much appreciated.

CHAPTER 1

Creating and Contesting Meaning in a Global Health Crisis

Ikuko Nakane, Claire Maree & Michael C. Ewing

Abstract

In response to disruptions during COVID-19, individuals and communities have creatively utilised discursive systems to navigate tense social atmospheres in the Asia-Pacific region. The interactions between layers of discursive practice are a crucial component of agentative meaning making which can facilitate contestation and inclusivity at local and national levels. In this introduction we map out the terrain of research to date, and identify the key themes which extend across the volume. Four "threads" which emerge from the exploration of discourses of disruption are woven together to present the key findings. These four threads are: discourses of disruption as sites of power struggle, impact of public discourse on social cohesion, contested meanings and identity, and intersections of language and culture.

Keywords: COVID-19, Asia, discourse and power, disruptions, national identity, crisis discourse

1. Communication in a Pandemic

The COVID-19 pandemic has brought about major shifts in the ways in which individuals, organisations, and nations operate in the world. As the virus spread through the globe, human movements were restricted and public health measures such as mask wearing and social distancing became the "new normal." Health authorities such as the World Health Organisation and disease control centres around the world issued updates and recommendations, leaders and governments engaged in public messaging to ensure proper implementation of public health measures, and individuals tried to make sense of what was happening by engaging with each other through social media and on- and off-line modes of contact. In a collective effort to contain this large-scale health emergency, communication has emerged as a crucial element of this disruptive global crisis.

In crisis situations, the meanings we create, and the way we create those meanings impact on the life and death of people. The primary aim of this volume is to highlight the centrality of communication in the face of such a global health crisis. Our focus is on the ways in which "disruptions" in relation to COVID-19 were created, addressed, and exacerbated in public discourse in Asian contexts.

COVID-19 has caused not only illness to individuals, but also disruptions to our health systems and social coherence. Public health communication therefore not only sought to contain the virus, but also to mitigate the other disruptions it has caused (O'Hair and O'Hair, 2021). The WHO and leaders around the world made appeals to the public through social media or press conferences to change their behaviour or routines in the hope of containing the virus, and government health departments continuously updated health directives on their websites to keep the public up to date on current best practice. The language of these directives was not merely instrumental; it was often aimed at creating a sense of solidarity in the face of threat, with a goal of bringing people together (Dada et al., 2021; Molnár, Takács, and Harnos, 2020).

While these communicative events were aimed at alleviating confusion and providing useful information, discourses of the pandemic and its impact have themselves created disruptions to social cohesion and further deepened the social divides which already existed. With these layers of disruption associated with COVID-19 in mind, the chapters in this volume offer insights into the various roles communication has played in public discourse, with a focus on the Asian region.

2. COVID-19 and Discourses of Disruption

Crisis comes in many different forms and is both "socially and discursively constructed" (De Rycker and Mohd Don, 2013, p. 10). The COVID-19 pandemic crisis has resulted in far-reaching large-scale disruptions. Health provision has been disrupted. Movement has been disrupted. Education and schooling have been disrupted. Work has been disrupted. Social and communal gatherings have been disrupted. All aspects of life and death, it could be argued, have been disrupted. COVID is, therefore, not only itself a disruption of physical health but also a cause of social disruption through which issues of power and agency come into focus in ways which have previously been obfuscated by "normativity" (cf. Coupland, 2020).

COVID-19 emerged in the era of widespread international interconnectivity, often referred to as globalisation. "Language-in-motion" is one resource for creating and understanding meaning within "various spatiotemporal frames interacting with one another" (Blommaert, 2010, p. 5). Blommaert argues for the importance of approaching language at "different, layered ... scale-levels." Scaling is, as Gal argues, "a relational practice that relies on situated comparisons among events, persons, and activities" (2016, p. 91). We scale by creating comparisons which extend over both space and time (Summerson, Carr, and Lempert, 2016). With digital connectivity a shared reality across the globe, and between private and public spaces, meaning is made and contested locally and globally from diverse perspectives using scales such as less/more, better/worse, equal/not equal and so on. In our inquiry into discourses of disruption, we cannot avoid the issue of mobility (and lack of it) and the inequalities it creates. However, as Dong (2021) suggests, the pause in global movement caused by the pandemic may require us to reconsider our conceptualisations of language in globalisation. To better understand discourses of disruption in COVID-19 as global, social, cultural, and political phenomena, this volume will attempt to unpack the multi-layered functioning of discursive resources.

3. Studies in Language and Discourse of COVID-19

Central to this volume is the examination of communication and language in the context of the COVID-19 global crisis as it unfolds in the Asia-Pacific. While the COVID-19 pandemic has been extensively studied from medical, public health and political perspectives, the crucial role of language and communication during the COVID crisis has received less attention. Of a number of key studies which have emerged in this area, several of those outlined here are related to the Asia region.

An early special issue of *Multilingua* (Piller, Zhang, and Li, 2020) focused on crisis communication in the Chinese context, including linguistically and culturally diverse communities within China as well as diasporic communities internationally, and with a focus on bringing peripheral academic voices into the global discourse. A close look at sociolinguistic research during the pandemic is presented by work in a special issue of *Linguistics Vanguard* (Sneller, 2022; Abtahian et al., 2022) on international students from East Asia and South Asia, focusing on ethical concerns related to researching personal experiences of the pandemic and looking for ways of improving public discourse during a crisis. More recently, the longer-term effects of COVID on national place branding have been investigated in a special issue of *Sociolinguistic Studies* (Tovar, 2023) with studies examining nationalistic governmental attempts to highlight their positive responses to the pandemic and promote tourism, but which can also engender negative reactions, resistance, and subversion from the public. These include case studies from Japan (Carlson and Hatano, 2023) and the Philippines (Vitorio and Valdez, 2023). Edited volumes have focused on humanities and social science perspectives, including pandemic crisis communication through journalism, literature, and advertising (Zhao et al., 2021, which includes several chapters on Chinese contexts) and problems arising specifically from translation and interpreting in both the Global North and Global

South (Blumczynski and Wilson, 2023; Liu and Cheung, 2022). The contributions in Musolff et al. (2022) examine discourses of public debate in several countries, reflecting on agenda setting, metaphor, and performativity by a wide range of actors, including those in Asia.

Chapters in the above-mentioned compilations, together with several individual studies, have highlighted a number of key themes arising from the study of language and communication during the pandemic, several of which are examined in chapters of this volume. Crisis and risk communications during the pandemic occur at a range of scales from the global to the national to the very local (Krystallidou and Braun, 2022). At the level of the nation state, in addition to public health messaging for their constituencies, governments have engaged in pandemic-inspired public relations campaigns. These involve biopolitical nationalism in East Asia (de Kloet and Lin, 2020) and place branding in Southeast Asia (Mathayomchan, Taecharungroj, and Wattanacharoensil, 2022), Japan, and the Philippines (Tovar, 2023), whereby nations promote their pandemic responses in a kind of nationalistic rivalry, to assert a positive global image, stimulate popular support, and revitalise tourism. Ideological responses to the pandemic have also influenced newspaper reporting and have been used in East Asia to attack international rivals and push for pro-business reforms (Fox, 2021).

A major issue originally identified by the World Health Organization during the SARS epidemic, and which became increasingly problematic during COVID-19, is what has been termed an "Infodemic" of misinformation and disinformation (Dang, 2021, on Southeast Asia; Dong, 2021, which includes the experience of migrant workers in China). Linguistically and culturally diverse communities are particularly vulnerable to such problems of communication (Krystallidou and Braun, 2022) and much of the research on language issues during the pandemic has centred on the needs of more marginalised communities. These are usually minority populations within societies dominated by a larger linguistic group, and they may be identified with indigenous languages (Sakhiyya et al., 2022 on Indonesia; Sengupta, 2022, which compares countries with high linguistic diversity including China, India, and Indonesia), the languages of permanent migrants, or of temporary visiting workers and students (Jang and Choi, 2020; Li et al., 2020). Many of the efforts to improve communication channels for marginalised groups have involved grassroots, bottom-up efforts by community members themselves. Zhang and Zhao (2020) have discussed vlogs in home languages, produced by Chinese YouTube micro-influencers living in the diaspora, as a way of communicating health messages to migrant communities. Indigenous Austronesian communities in Taiwan took it upon themselves to develop their own public health messaging campaigns in local languages, in the face of primarily Mandarin-language messaging from the government (Chen, 2020). Indeed, volunteer translating and interpreting initiatives have been developed by many local and migrant communities to fill the gap left by inadequate government information programmes, as evidenced in the examples from China (Jiang, 2021; Zhang and Wu, 2020; Zheng, 2020). One cause of this inadequacy in some jurisdictions has been an English-mediated multilingualism, which assumes that English is the default "foreign" language and is mistakenly believed to be adequate for communicating with migrants from a variety of linguistic backgrounds—an issue identified in, for example, China (Jiang, 2021; Li et al., 2020; Zheng, 2020) and Japan (Nakamura, 2022). Due to these problems, there is a noted increase in the valorisation of minority languages (e.g., Bai, 2020 on Inner-Mongolia, China; Li et al., 2020 on China) along with a call for greater government support for marginalised language communities (Chen, 2020 on Taiwan; Heinrichs, Kretzer, and Davis, 2022 on Australia; Jang and Choi, 2020 and Shen, 2020 on China; Sengupta, 2022 on several countries including China, India, and Indonesia).

These bottom-up efforts contrast with frequently less effective top-down government approaches. Public health messages may be ineffectual when the language proficiencies of the general population are not considered by governments, as Sakhiyya et al. (2022) argue based on their study in Indonesia. On the other hand, uncritical translation into migrant languages can also have a negative impact: Chesnut, Curran, and Kim (2023) show that the choice of languages for the translation of government public signage in Korea is based on stereotypes about perceived behaviours by specific migrant groups; this in turn reinforces these negative stereotypes in the broader community. Nonetheless, the power and resources held by governments make them vital players in public health communication, and key themes to emerge are the importance of support from authorities for grassroots efforts and the need for all actors to look for coproduced solutions (Jang and Choi, 2020 on South Korea; Krystallidou and Braun, 2022 covering several jurisdictions including China and Taiwan).

In sum, there is an increasing volume of studies on language and communication related to COVID-19, covering a range of areas such as multilingual communication, linguistic minority communities, translation and interpreting, public health communication, media discourse, and language and national identity. Chapters in this volume also cover these areas of inquiry, with a specific focus on how people, media, organisations, and governments dealt with the extraordinary challenges of disruptions posed by COVID-19 through their meaning-making activities in Asian languages. The contributors to this volume, all of whom have expertise in Asian studies, bring much-needed insight to discourses of the pandemic beyond the Anglophone world.

4. Overview of the Volume

The chapters in this book focus on the multiple disruptions to people (individuals), entities, and governments in the Asian region where a "new normal" has brought into question "normality." These ongoing disruptions affect shared community values, human rights, and everyday activities. At first constructed as "unexpected," to those not in the relevant fields of epidemiology, COVID-19 disruptions have controlled narratives in public discourse. Since early 2020, this ongoing state of disruption has become normalised.

The contributions to this volume are set within scholarship from disciplines such as Asian studies, translation studies, sociolinguistics, and discourse analysis. The individual chapters examine media flows, public discourse, and issues of translation. Using diverse approaches to, and issues regarding, languages in societies from the Asian region, the chapters explore the struggles over national identity and manifestations of socio-political issues in the context of disruptions caused by the ongoing COVID-19 pandemic. Methodologies include discourse analysis, sociolinguistics of stance, pragmatics, and translation studies. Data derive from public discourses in Cantonese, Chinese, Japanese, Korean, Malay, and Australian English. The types of texts under scrutiny in this volume range from news articles and official government announcements to social media posts by the general public.

In Chapter 2, Susanna Ackroyd provides insight into how the Communist Party of China (CPC) constructs and manages discourse around public health crises such as the SARS and COVID-19 pandemics. Specifically, using a Critical Discourse Analysis approach, this chapter examines how the CPC employs a battle-hero-saviour narrative to leverage the Party's revolutionary history and strengthen the legitimacy of its rule, thus informing the larger story of Chinese governance and nation-building under the CPC.

The pandemic has also revealed challenges of public health communication in the era of globalisation. Since timeliness of communication is crucial in order to avoid further disruptions to health crisis management, government agencies have become increasingly dependent on machine translation. Examining the performance of Neural Machine Translation (NMT) tools in translating Chinese language journal articles about COVID-19, Wayne Wen-chun Liang, Ester S.M. Leung, and Chun Hin Tse in Chapter 3 identify what MT evaluation metrics fail to reflect in the quality of translation, while also presenting a refined set of quality assessment metrics to explore how the evaluation of machine-translated texts can better be undertaken. The chapter highlights the importance of cultural, emotional, or ideological dimensions when communicating across languages.

The public health emergency of COVID-19 brought disruptions not only to the everyday lives of the citizens, but also to the 2020 Olympic and Paralympic Games. In

Chapter 4, Claire Maree explores how disruptions caused by the ongoing COVID-19 pandemic created tensions and clashes with the 2020 Tokyo Olympic Games' vision of "Unity in Diversity" and "United by Emotion," as seen in increasing xenophobia and protest against the Games. It is argued that the polite undertones of おもてなし [omotenashi] (selfless hospitality) resonate with the impolite demands to "get out" in a way that demonstrates the fragility of omotenashi as an act of un/welcoming the foreign.

Turning to the disruptions which threaten the effort to unite a nation to fight against the pandemic, Ikuko Nakane focuses on efforts to stop discrimination due to COVID-19. This chapter discusses discursive resources and underlying ideological stances of the producer of public messages against coronavirus discrimination. The analysis reveals intersecting layers of discourses which emerge from the different socio-political positionings of the creators of these messages. Along with Susanna Ackroyd's chapter, Nakane's chapter demonstrates how the "war" metaphor is used as a powerful tool for health crisis management, but at the same time may obscure underlying problems in the society.

Chapter 6 further explores the issue of social tension caused by the pandemic. Jun Ohashi examines how perceived social norms and moral concerns for self and others have shaped the discourses and practices of mask wearing during the COVID-19 pandemic. Focusing on how social norms and social identities are formed in online discussion forums in Japan and in Australia, the chapter argues that the topic of (non-)mask wearing provides interesting material for the study of interpersonal language and (im)politeness.

Mi Yung Park and Hakyoon Lee in Chapter 7 present the unexpected impact of the disruption which COVID-19 brought to the increasingly multicultural and multilingual Korean society. The chapter discusses how bilingual and bicultural capacities of marginalised minority women in South Korea give them agency in contributing to public health initiatives. Importantly, it is argued that the women's contribution amidst the nation's struggles with COVID-19 has impacted upon the discourses of identity politics.

In Chapter 8, Richard Powell and Zarina Othman examine discourses of "confusion" found in reports and in reader comments in the online news portal *Malaysiakini*, focusing on uncertainty about COVID-19 containment measures. Employing a Critical Discourse Analysis framework to explore the stances behind these discourses, the chapter argues that such confusion concerns how such orders and procedures are communicated, while also indexing political frustration and dissatisfaction with the health measures themselves.

In Chapter 9, Craig A. Smith and Dayton Lekner examine how one of the key binaries of Chinese thought—that of 內–外 [nei–wai] (internal–external)—has evolved in Taiwan during the COVID-19 pandemic and is reflected in its discourses on its neighbours. The chapter argues that the pandemic has served as a meta-catalyst in which material and discursive conditions continue to transform the way that Taiwanese construct and understand their identity and their place in the world.

Finally, in Chapter 10 Lachlan Thomas-Walters, Suqin Qian, and Delia Lin highlight the complexity of communicating public health information to culturally and linguistically diverse communities. This chapter argues that quality translation is the foundation of the coherent and well-informed approach to communication which responsible government bodies owe linguistic minorities in times of health emergency.

The overarching theme of "discourses of disruption," therefore, emerges from interdisciplinary and intradisciplinary collaboration between the authors. It addresses the multiplicity of communication modes and mediums which are critical in the management of public health crises, and the ways in which these are impacted on by social, political, and cultural fissures.

5. Emerging Threads of Discourses of Disruption in Asia: Creating and Contesting Meaning in the Time of COVID-19

This edited volume focuses on the earlier stages of the COVID-19 pandemic, reflecting on 2020 to mid-2021, not the "COVID normal" third year phase. Four **threads** emerge from the study of *Discourses of Disruption in Asia: Creating and Contesting Meaning in the Time of COVID-19* in this earlier stage and in the context of the Asia-Pacific and languages from the region: sites of power struggle, disruptions to social cohesion, contested meanings, and intersections of language and culture.

5.1 Thread 1: Sites of Power Struggle

Communication is central in times of disruption. The chapters in this volume offer an analysis of a variety of texts—newspaper articles, journal articles, medical texts, official government announcements, health directives, comments by the "general public" on social media apps and comments by civil society actors—which offer alternatives to Anglo-European perspectives of the pandemic. When compiled, the analysis of this wide variety of texts demonstrates how public discourse emerges as a site for power struggle where, for example, governments attempt to implement measures to contain the disease. In Ackroyd's story grammar analysis of the *People's Daily* newspaper and Nakane's discussion of government leaders' video messages against "corona discrimination," the "war" metaphor emerges as a discursive resource to mobilise and unite the nation against a disease which could disrupt not only the health system but also trust in the government. Public discourses on

COVID-19 also emerge as a site for power struggle in relation to geopolitical conflicts in the Asia-Pacific. Polarised "us and them" positioning over the handling of the health crisis is illustrated by the discussion of antagonistic voices in traditional and social media in Taiwan (Chapter 9, Smith and Lekner).

The discourses of COVID-19 disruption have also created a space for the public to express their discontent with authorities, threatening the authorities' power and control. Maree's discussion of contrastive おもてなし [*omotenashi*] (Japanese hospitality) and 帰れ [*kaere*] (go home!) discourses highlight the dynamic workings of linguistic politeness in Japanese in the articulation of dissent against the power holders, illustrating disruption to the management of a global event in the midst of a pandemic. In Powell and Othman's chapter, the analysis of the news media discourse in Malaysia sheds light on how the public might capitalise on the discourse of confusion over the communication of public health regulations to express their discontent and opposition to the government. Powell and Othman also argue that inability to avoid confusion creates a challenging context for power struggle, especially if the authority is regarded as "untrustworthy" or "incompetent." Such research explicates how discursive resources are deployed by nations and governments, not only to protect their people from the virus but also to maintain their power during a significant health crisis which presented an opening for potential disruptions to the regime. Indeed, studies in this volume demonstrate that discursive strategies with varying modalities are adopted by citizens and journalists and at times even threaten a regime's control of its political power.

5.2 Thread 2: Disruptions to Social Cohesion

A second key thread which emerges from the work presented in this volume points to how public discourse contributed to disruptions to social cohesion, creating, exacerbating, or reconfiguring social tensions and discrimination. Ohashi's analysis of public forum discussions on mask wearing in Japan and Australia reveals new social tensions arising as people expressed their stances towards public health measures and expected behaviour. In the Japanese forum, norm-conforming pressure resulted in aggressive and impolite language used against the opposing group in Japan, while solidarity-oriented discourse prevailed over willingness to conform to the new norm of mask wearing in the Australian forum. This highlights tensions over normative behaviour and illustrates how discourse on such behavioural norms is enacted in digital spaces.

Disruption to social cohesion has also manifested itself in rising discrimination against people who contracted COVID-19—even essential workers, including health workers. While we have seen public displays of support for health workers and calls for solidarity in many parts of the world, governments, health authorities such as WHO, and human rights groups also launched campaigns against discrimination associated with COVID-19. Nakane's chapter reveals a range of linguistic and semiotic resources which Japanese leaders used to address a threat to social cohesion driven by discrimination. Their varying approaches have implications for effective leadership communication in times of national and global crisis.

Public discourse on COVID-19 has also been discussed as a locus for exclusion and inclusion of minority groups. The pandemic has resulted in exclusion of linguistic minorities due to lack of access to quality services and information (Piller, Zhang, and Li, 2020). A pitfall of multilingual policy in the health crisis context is closely examined by Thomas-Walters, Qian and Lin in their study of multilingual public health communication. Contradictory consequences of exclusion and inclusion in public health translation practice emerge in their study, whereby the authorities' aspiration to be inclusive by providing multilingual information on COVID-19 public health measures falls short at times, as poor-quality translation entails risks of miscommunication, potentially causing disruption to social cohesion.

In the cases of Taiwan and Korea, contradictions are found when discourses of integration and inclusion are scrutinised in relation to the pandemic's disruptions. Smith and Lekner argue that there is a disjuncture highlighted in the scaling of discourse around the pandemic in that Taiwan's New Southbound Policy rhetoric of collaboration with Asia does not align with the prevalent portrayal of Southeast Asian migrant workers as outsiders in traditional and social media. Nor does it align with their exclusion from the information network. Smith and Lekner also contend that Taiwan's public discourse projects conflicting positionings vis-à-vis the international community over its positive COVID-19 management. Park and Lee's chapter also focuses on exclusion and inclusion, critically addressing social tension in the context of *wuli* (we) discourse. Their analysis of personal narratives of migrant women in newspaper articles illustrates how the disruptions to daily activities in a host community due to COVID-19 restrictions affected the women's sense of belonging and opportunities to be part of the community. Of particular interest here are the evolving and at times contradictory roles of migrant wives' bilingualism/biculturalism in the "new normal" context of the pandemic in Korea.

5.3 Thread 3: Contested Meanings

The work in this volume presents examples of how "crises and conflicts (like wars) play an important role in the formation and discursive construction of identities" (De Rycker and Mohd Don, 2013, p. 40). Contestations of meanings intensified as nations, governments, and individuals faced the challenges of shifting dynamics in the world around them caused by the pandemic. Intersecting with these social divisions is the issue of identity.

One of the subthemes of identity highlighted in this volume is that of national or regional identity. Through manipulating these conceptualisations of identity, a governing authority sets itself apart from others in its public discourse, describing its own nation or region as superior to others in their management of the health crisis. Examples from the *People's Daily* discussed by Ackroyd illustrate how China is portrayed as a successful leader in the international community in opposition to the negative image of the U.S. On the other hand, Taiwanese public discourse distanced itself from the PRC, capitalising on its own (initial) success in managing COVID-19 and othering the mainland Chinese community (Smith and Lekner). Taiwan's paradoxical identity positioning also played out in the public discourse which indulged in negative stereotyping of nationalities in their handling of the disease.

The health crisis has also highlighted how the agency of different groups of people intersected with the power endowed by linguistic repertoire. The analysis of news articles on foreign marriage-migrant women in Korea (Park and Lee) reveals that their cultural and linguistic minority status could lead to two contrary perceptions of their identity: valuable multilingual/multicultural members of mainstream Korean society who actively make positive contributions to society, or powerless and incompetent women who are a burden on its prosperity.

The COVID-19 pandemic has not only reconfigured identity positioning or intensified existing "us and them" discourse, but has also generated identity categories built on orientation to health measures and the disease. This is illustrated by the study of social media discourse on masks (Ohashi), where "pro-masker" and "anti-masker" identities were constructed through various discursive resources. There are other types of newly emerging identity categories associated with COVID-19 such as "pro-vaxxer" and "anti-vaxxer" which deserve future investigation from discourse perspectives.

5.4 Thread 4: Intersections of Language and Culture

Chapters in this volume demonstrate the significance of the complex and nuanced ways in which language and culture intersect in understanding discourses of COVID-19 disruption. The two chapters addressing translation issues (Thomas-Walters, Qian, and Lin; Liang, Leung, and Tse) identify layers of meaning embedded in the cultural and historical context of health-related communication, and highlight the challenges of ensuring effective and inclusive translation practice in culturally and linguistically diverse communities at the time of a global health crisis. The volume also touches upon an interesting aspect of multilingual communication, namely code-mixing, which is a discursive resource for both the making and the contestation of meaning, as discussed by Nakane, and by Powell and Othman.

Cultural terms which are grounded in specific sociolinguistic contexts are also used to both make and contest meaning. For example, the Japanese terms *meiwaku* (annoying) (Ohashi) or *omotenashi* (selfless hospitality) (Maree), and the caricaturised descriptions of how people from other nations handled the pandemic (Smith and Lekner), are drawn upon as powerful drivers of discourse which provide relevant sociocultural contexts of the discourses of disruption beyond the health crisis itself. This focus on the intersection of language and culture allows our work to move between etic and emic perspectives, in our attempt to capture how discourse operates at different scale-levels.

6. Creating and Contesting Meaning through Asian Languages

COVID is in and of itself a disruptive disease which causes physical and material harm to the individual body. These bodies are also "containers" through which the disease is distributed, hence the limits placed on both domestic and international movement. At local and global levels (cf. De Rycker and Mohd Don, 2013) governments and regimes have been invested in controlling the discourse of disruption as well as controlling disruptions to dominant discourse.

Communication of disruption has been essential to ensuring the ongoing functioning of local communities, regions, and countries. At the local level, individuals require details of what and how their everyday lives are to be affected by public health measures. At the same time, this volume highlights communication *as* disruption, where it has itself caused further disturbance due to a perceived lack of clarity, or unintentional misreading. As there are multifaceted individual and/ or institutional goals in addressing disruption, these often reinforce social norms, regimes of discrimination, and social injustices, the effects of which are diverse and intersectional.

Disruption causes both material and affective responses. The material effects of misinformation, for example, can lead to issues in accessing healthcare and essential services. A multiplicity of affective responses to that disruption can lead to, for example, feelings of frustration, grief, anger, or confusion. Due to such material and affective repercussions, the pandemic has tested the trust and confidence the public place in their government and political leaders. The actions and messaging of local leadership came under constant public scrutiny, not only because the nature of the new virus was unknown and confusing information circulated widely, but also because the threat of the new virus amplified pre-pandemic tension amongst socially divided public opinions about governance. Uncertainty and fear over a newly discovered health threat caused tension and conflicts in communication.

Social media platforms and spaces emerged as key sites of contestation and negotiation of meaning. SNS channels offered individuals opportunities to seek information online and also to express their opinions, instantly accessible by millions of others.

The pandemic also gave rise to redefinitions of national and regional identities. The discourse of "us vs them" became visible soon after a new coronavirus was identified and its first outbreak in Wuhan was reported. As cases spread around the world, racism against Chinese people began to rise as the virus was called the "Wuhan virus" or the "China virus" (Vazquez, 2020) with a xenophobic tone. "Discourses of disruption" associated with the pandemic, then, also cause disruption to social structures, human relations, and existing ideologies about them both. One of the key concerns of this volume, therefore, is to address how identities are redefined through discourses of the pandemic as a disruption and as a cause of disruptions. Gallois and Liu (2021) also warn of social and individual in addition to health consequences if the diverse orientations of the population within the community are not taken into account. By focusing on alternative discourses, power structures and social norms are brought into relief.

In the evolving context of the "new normal" of the pandemic, public discourses became a locus of contestations which generated further disruptions such as discrimination, reconfiguration of identities, and power struggles. This volume of work explores the impact of COVID-19, unpacking it from a combination of local meaning-making perspectives and wider sociocultural perspectives. The multiple perspectives outlined in this volume enable us to explore complex and multifaceted roles of communication as disruptions are created and circulated throughout the global community. The contributors' translingual and transcultural lenses bring to light how communities around Asia made sense of the monumental challenges posed by the pandemic from inside and outside. Our work aims to show that discourses of disruption do not necessarily entail negative consequences, but can give new openings for contesting and making meanings to reimagine the world around us. The work in this book focuses on public discourse to complement studies of discourse on and of COVID-19 in other genres and thus to further our understanding of health crisis communication.

The COVID-19 pandemic has gone through a number of phases since the virus was first reported in 2020. This project does not include discussion of discourse on COVID-19 vaccination or easing of restrictions beyond the third year of the pandemic. Given the centrality of language and communication in this global health crisis, further investigation of disruptions in these new phases of the pandemic from discourse perspectives will have important implications, not only for public health but also for solidarity of, and hope for, humanity.

Ikuko Nakane is Associate Professor in Japanese at the University of Melbourne. Her research interests include sociolinguistics, discourse analysis, multilingualism, and legal discourse. Her work primarily focuses on negotiation of power and solidarity in institutional discourse. Her articles have appeared in journals such as *Journal of Pragmatics, Semiotica,* and *Multilingua.*

Claire Maree is Professor in Japanese, Asia Institute, University of Melbourne. A queer theorist and linguist, Claire Maree mobilises linguistic and cultural studies methodologies to examine language, identity, and the media. Claire's work has been foundational to the establishment of Japanese language, gender, and sexuality studies.

Michael C. Ewing is Associate Professor in Indonesian Studies, University of Melbourne. Michael's research interests include interactional linguistics and linguistic anthropology, with a focus on the languages of Indonesia. His current work involves the youth language and the nexus between standard and colloquial modes of grammatical organisation in everyday conversation.

References

Abtahian, Maya Ravindranath, Naomi Nagy, Katharina Pabst, and Vidhya Elango. 2022. "Disruptions due to COVID-19: Using mixed methods to identify factors influencing language maintenance and shift." *Linguistics Vanguard* 8, no. s3: 331–341. https://doi.org/10.1515/lingvan-2021-0057.

Bai, Gogentuul Hongye. 2020. "Fighting COVID-19 with Mongolian fiddle stories." *Multilingua* 39, no. 5: 577–586.

Blommaert, Jan. 2010. *The Sociolinguistics of Globalization.* Cambridge: Cambridge University Press. doi:10.1017/CBO9780511845307

Blumczynski, Piotr, and Steven Wilson, eds. 2023. *The Languages of COVID-19: Translational and Multilingual Perspectives on Global Healthcare.* New York: Routledge.

Carlson, Rebecca, and Hiroto Hatano. 2023. "Branding a pandemic response: The biopolitics of (marketing) infection control in Japan." *Sociolinguistics Studies* 16, no. 4: 485–503.

Chen, Chun-Mei. 2020. "Public health messages about COVID-19 prevention in multilingual Taiwan." *Multilingua* 39, no. 5: 597–606. https://doi.org/10.1515/multi-2020-0092.

Chesnut, Michael, Nathaniel Ming Curran, and Sungwoo Kim. 2023. "From garbage to COVID-19: Theorizing 'Multilingual Commanding Urgency' in the linguistic landscape." *Multilingua* 42 no. 1: 25–53.

Coupland, Nik. 2020. Normativity, Language & COVID-19. *Working Papers in Urban Language & Literacies* no. 271.

Dada, Sara, Henry Charles Ashworth, Marlene Joannie Bewa, and Roopa Dhatt. 2021. "Words matter: Political and gender analysis of speeches made by heads of government during the COVID-19 pandemic." *BMJ Global Health* 6: e003910.

Dang, Hoang Linh. 2021. "Social media, fake news, and the COVID-19 pandemic: Sketching the case of Southeast Asia." *Austrian Journal of South-East Asian Studies* 14, no. 1: 37–57.

de Kloet, Jeroen, and Jian Lin. 2020. "'We are doing better': Biopolitical nationalism and the COVID-19 virus in East Asia." *European Journal of Cultural Studies* 23, no. 4: 635–640.

De Rycker, Antoon, and Zuraidah Mohd Don. 2013. "Discourse in crisis, crisis in discourse." In *Discourse and Crisis: Critical Perspectives*, edited by Antoon De Rycker and Zuraidah Mohd Don, 3–65. Amsterdam: John Benjamins Publishing Company.

Dong, Jie. 2021. "Language and globalization revisited: Life from the periphery in COVID-19." *International Journal of the Sociology of Language* 2021, no. 267-268: 105–110. https://doi.org/10.1515/ijsl-2020-0086.

Fox, Colm A. 2021. "Media in a time of crisis: Newspaper coverage of COVID-19 in East Asia." *Journalism Studies* 22, no. 13: 1853–1873.

Gallois, Cindy, and Shuang Liu. 2021. "Power and the pandemic: A perspective from communication and social psychology." *Journal of Multicultural Discourses* 16, no.1: 20–26.

Heinrichs, Danielle H., Michael M. Kretzer, and Emily E. Davis. 2022. "Mapping the online language ecology of multilingual COVID-19 public health information in Australia." *European Journal of Language Policy* 14, no. 2: 133–162.

Jang, In Chull, and Lee Jin Choi. 2020. "Staying connected during COVID-19: The social and communicative role of an ethnic online community of Chinese international students in South Korea." *Multilingua* 39, no. 5: 541–552. https://doi.org/10.1515/multi-2020-0097.

Jiang, Mengying. 2021. "Translating against COVID-19 in the Chinese context: A multi-agent, multimedia and multilingual endeavor." In *COVID-19 Pandemic, Crisis Responses and the Changing World: Perspectives in Humanities and Social Sciences*, edited by Simon X.B. Zhao, Johnston H.C. Wong, Charles Lowe, Edoardo Monaco, and John Corbett, 229–241. Singapore: Springer.

Krystallidou, Demi, and Sabine Braun. 2022. "Risk and crisis communication during COVID-19 in linguistically and culturally diverse communities: A scoping review of the available evidence." In *The Languages of COVID-19: Translational and Multilingual Perspectives on Global Healthcare*, edited by Piotr Blumczynski and Steven Wilson, 128–144. New York: Routledge.

Li, Jia, Ping Xie, Bin Ai, and Lisheng Li. 2020. "Multilingual communication experiences of international students during the COVID-19 Pandemic." *Multilingua* 39, no. 5: 529–539. https://doi.org/10.1515/multi-2020-0116.

Liu, Kanglong and Andrew K. F. Cheung, eds. 2022. *Translation and Interpreting in the Age of COVID-19*. Singapore: Springer.

Mathayomchan, Boonyanit, Viriya Taecharungroj, and Walanchalee Wattanacharoensil. 2022. "Evolution of COVID-19 tweets about Southeast Asian Countries: Topic modelling and sentiment analyses." *Place Branding and Public Diplomacy* 19: 317–334. https://doi.org/10.1057/s41254-022-00271-5.

Molnár, Anna, Lili Takács, and Éva Jakusné Harnos. 2020. "Securitization of the COVID-19 pandemic by metaphoric discourse during the State of Emergency in Hungary." *International Journal of Sociology and Social Policy* 40, no. 9/10: 1167–1182.

Musolff, Andreas, Ruth Breeze, Kayo Kondo, and Sara Vilar-Lluch, eds. (2022). *Pandemic and Crisis Discourse: Communicating COVID-19 and Public Health Strategy*. London: Bloomsbury Academic.

Nakamura, Janice. 2022. "COVID-19 signs in Tokyo and Kanagawa: Linguistic landscaping for whom?" *Asia-Pacific Social Science Review* 22, no. 30: 80–94.

O'Hair, H. Dan, and Mary John O'Hair. 2021. "Managing science communication in a pandemic." In *Communicating Science in Times of Crisis: COVID-19 Pandemic*, edited by H. Dan O'Hair and Mary John O'Hair, 3–14. Hoboken, NJ: John Wiley & Sons.

Piller, Ingrid., Jie Zhang, and Jia Li. 2020. "Linguistic diversity in a time of crisis: Language challenges of the COVID-19 pandemic." *Multilingua*, 39, no. 5: 503–515. http://dx.doi.org/10.1515/multi-2020-0136.

Sakhiyya, Zulfa, Girindra Putri Dewi Saraswati, Zuhrul Anam, and Abdul Azis. 2022. "What's in a name? Crisis communication during the COVID-19 pandemic in multilingual Indonesia." *International Journal of Multilingualism*. https://doi.org/10.1080/14790718.2022.2127732.

Sengupta, Papia. 2022. "Language, communication, and the COVID-19 pandemic: Criticality of multi-lingual education." *International Journal of Multilingualism:* 1–14, https://doi.org/10.1080/14790718.2021.2021918.

Shen, Qi. 2020. "Commentary: Directions in language planning from the COVID-19 pandemic." *Multilingua* 39, no. 5: 625–629. https://doi.org/10.1515/multi-2020-0133.

Sneller, Betsy. 2022. "COVID-era sociolinguistics: Introduction to the special issue." *Linguistics Vanguard* 8, no. s3: 303–306. https://doi.org/10.1515/lingvan-2021-0138.

Summerson Carr, E., and Michael Lepmert. 2016. *Scale: Discourse and Dimensions of Social Life.* Berkeley: University of California Press. https://doi.org/10.1515/9780520965430.

Tovar, Johanna. 2023. "The role of language in place branding during the Covid-19 pandemic and post-lockdowns: An introduction." *Sociolinguistic Studies* 16, no. 4: 423–433. https://doi.org/10.1558/sols.23528.

Vazquez, Marietta. 2020. "Calling COVID-19 the 'Wuhan Virus' or 'China Virus' is inaccurate and xenophobic." *Yale School of Medicine*, March 12, 2020. https://medicine.yale.edu/news-article/calling-covid-19-the-wuhan-virus-or-china-virus-is-inaccurate-and-xenophobic/.

Vitorio, Raymund, and Paolo Niño Valdez. 2023. "The taming of the shrewd: Technologies of the self, emotions, and the rebranding of Philippine tourism." *Sociolinguistic Studies* 16, no. 4: 505–524. https://doi.org/10.1558/sols.23527.

Zhang, Jie, and Yuqin Wu. 2020. "Providing multilingual logistics communication in COVID-19 disaster relief." *Multilingua* 39, no. 5: 517–528. https://doi.org/10.1515/multi-2020-0110.

Zhang, Leticia-Tian and Sumin Zhao. 2020. "Diaspora micro-influencers and COVID-19 communication on social media: The case of Chinese-speaking YouTube vloggers." *Multilingua* 39, no. 5, 553–563. https://doi.org/10.1515/multi-2020-0099.

Zhao, Simon X.B., Johnston H.C. Wong, Charles Lowe, Edoardo Monaco, and John Corbett, eds. 2021. *COVID-19 Pandemic, Crisis Responses and the Changing World: Perspectives in Humanities and Social Sciences.* Singapore: Springer.

Zheng, Yongyan. 2020. "Mobilizing foreign language students for multilingual crisis translation in Shanghai." *Multilingua* 39, no. 5: 587–595. https://doi.org/10.1515/multi-2020-0095.

CHAPTER 2

Martyrs in Masks: the "Battle-Hero-Saviour" Story Grammar of COVID-19 Coverage in Chinese Communist Party Media

Susanna Ackroyd

Abstract

Using a Critical Discourse Analysis approach, this chapter provides insight into how the Communist Party of China (CPC) constructs and manages discourse around public health crises. Specifically, how the CPC employed a battle-hero-saviour narrative during the initial COVID-19 outbreak in Wuhan to leverage the Party's revolutionary history and strengthen the legitimacy of its rule, thus informing the larger story of Chinese governance and nation-building under the CPC.

Keywords: Chinese Communist Party media, battle-hero-saviour narrative, crisis response, Chinese governance, nation-building

The disruption brought by the COVID-19 pandemic has both challenged and further legitimised the Communist Party of China (CPC). Domestically, the initial outbreak in 2020 resulted in mass shutdowns and harsh restrictions being imposed upon hundreds of millions of people, including a seventy-six-day total lockdown in Wuhan. It also served as a double-edged sword for China on the international stage—much criticism was directed at the Chinese government for its initial response, but it provided an opportunity for authoritarian China to demonstrate its (initial) success in controlling the spread of the disease and its willingness as a major international power to cooperate with other countries in the provision of aid and medical expertise. Through Critical Discourse Analysis of coverage of the pandemic in the *People's Daily*, this chapter argues that the CPC has shaped the discourse of COVID-19 in domestic media to strengthen its political legitimacy by employing a set pattern of three distinct, recurring, and intertwined narratives:

- that the anti-pandemic effort is a battle against the enemy of COVID-19 (*battle*)
- that frontline workers are heroic soldiers fighting on that battlefield (*hero*)
- that only under the leadership of the Communist Party of China can an ultimate victory be assured (*saviour*)

The research in this chapter has analysed Chinese-language articles from the *People's Daily* from the first mention of COVID-19 in January 2020 and through the height of the initial outbreak until May 2020, when control was achieved and coverage shifted away from immediate response measures. Newspaper articles were gathered either directly from the official website of the *People's Daily* newspaper (paper.people.com.cn) or via the China National Knowledge Infrastructure database. Quotations from the *People's Daily* in this chapter have been translated into English by the author. In-text citations are attributed to the article's listed authors; where no author is presented, the source is cited as *People's Daily*.

The 人民日报 [*Renmin Ribao*] (herein: *People's Daily*) is the official newspaper of the Central Committee of the Communist Party of China and is formally the highest organ of the Party outside of the National Party Congresses which are held every five years. It has a current circulation of 3 million (People's Daily Online, n.d.). According to the *People's Daily*'s self-profile, for more than seventy years the newspaper has served to actively promote the Party's theories, principles, policies, and major decisions. Since entering the 21st Century, it has been led by Deng Xiaoping Theory and Xi Jinping Thought to firmly guide 'correct public opinion' 正确舆论 [*zhengque yulun*], publicise the deeds of both Party cadres and the masses, and proudly lead the country to triumph in revolution, construction, and reform (People's Daily Online, n.d.).

Though the *People's Daily* is a newspaper, it is not a vehicle for disseminating news; rather it is a tool to propagate ideology from the Party elite. The *People's Daily* and other Party publications interpret the world and shape discourse from the view of the elite of the CPC, maintaining a classic propaganda function of the press while also guiding the general direction of private commercial media outlets (Wang, Sparks, and Huang, 2018).

1. Background: Narratives of War and Heroes in Communist China

Official CPC discourse around China's modern history contains "national narratives" (Gries, 2007, p. 114) of crisis and war threatening the nation, with the Party ultimately saving China. The most well-known example of this is the "Century of Humiliation" narrative, referring to the period of Chinese history from the Opium Wars and the loss of Hong Kong and Macau to colonial powers, through the Japanese invasion and occupation of mainland China up until the founding of the People's Republic of China in 1949 (Gries, 2007, p. 116). The Century of Humiliation discourse presents pre-CPC China as fractured and feeble, and the narrative of humiliation by foreign powers and subsequent rejuvenation of China resonates in present day via the Chinese government's patriotic education campaign, which aims to tie the

Party's legitimacy to nationalist sentiment following the increasing irrelevance of Communist ideology in the post-reform era (Zhao, 1998).

In both the revolutionary era and post-reform China, official narratives simplify and distil these events and their actors into a Manichean war of "good" versus "evil." That is not to say they are wholly invented—Gries (2007) argues that official narratives of Chinese history are neither totally objective nor wholly invented by the CPC as a political tool, but rather that an interactive relationship between the Party-State and bottom-up nationalism shapes how stories of China's past are understood, presented and even challenge CPC governance. Nevertheless, in official narratives the Communist Party is presented as good and righteous (Gries, 2007, p. 116). These narratives not only assert the success and strength of the CPC, but also establish an understanding of Communist Party leadership as integral to the continued success of the People's Republic of China. To support the Communist Party is to support China; to be a nationalist is to be loyal to the CPC, as without the CPC there would be no China.

The CPC uses individual heroes in these narratives as models to reiterate ideal relations between the Party and the people, and aid in shaping citizens' behaviour and solidarity in a way which strengthens Party rule. The use of models in modern Chinese governance is the continuity of a Confucian cultural tradition adopted by the CPC in the revolutionary era, and its resilience as a discourse practice underlines its usefulness in maintaining social control. Bakken argues that "one of the fundamental assumptions in the Chinese theory of learning [is] that people are innately capable of learning from models" (2000, p. 8). In the Mao era, the Communist Party promoted several heroic servicemen as models for its citizenry, with Lei Feng the most well known.

An orphan rescued by the Party in a nascent People's Republic of China, official history records Lei Feng as altruistic and selflessly devoted to progression of the revolution under Mao Zedong's leadership; he diligently washed his comrades' bedding and rinsed cabbages to feed officers and recruits to support the cause. Lei Feng died in 1962, aged in his early twenties, after being "martyred" by a telephone pole knocked over by a reversing army truck. Following his death, his personal diary became an important source of propaganda for the Communist Party and the "Learn from Comrade Lei Feng" campaign encouraged Chinese citizens to emulate his behaviour. In his diary he wrote of his selfless deeds, his admiration and reverence of Mao and his desire to function as "a screw that never rusts" within the revolutionary machinery (Edwards, 2010; Jeffreys and Su, 2016).

Official narratives of Chinese history glorify those who quietly, and without seeking outside praise, complete the necessary but unglamorous tasks required to carry forward the aims of the Party with unwavering loyalty and self-sacrifice. Lei Feng's value to the CPC as a model is not derived from military heroism or wartime achievement—his death was not the result of some heroic gesture, but rather an unimpressive accident. The value of his story (as well as the stories of other "model servicemen" promoted by the Party, including Ouyang Hai and Wang Jie) comes from Lei Feng's blind devotion to the Party, contentment to function as a small part of a greater whole, and willingness to sacrifice himself for the good of the revolution. This theme has continued into contemporary Party-society relations.

2. Findings: The Battle-Hero-Saviour Story Grammar

The *People's Daily* frames China's efforts to control and eliminate COVID-19 in terms of warfare, invoking historical narratives of struggle against enemies to position the CPC as a constant saviour of the Chinese people and reinforce its leadership as integral to the nation's continued survival. It transforms revolutionary heroes into social models, establishing an expectation of individual sacrifice for the public good, and provides a justification for otherwise unreasonable demands. Through this, the Party moulds discourse around COVID-19 to strengthen its position as the paramount authority in China.

Coverage of COVID-19 in the *People's Daily* follows a "battle-hero-saviour" story grammar—that is, a meta-narrative with three components. Each component consists of its own narrative which can be extracted and employed alone, or alongside either (or both) of the other parts. The following sections of this chapter analyse coverage of COVID-19 through a framework structured around this story grammar.

The structure of multiple parallel and intertwined narratives as a "story grammar" and its related analytical framework draw inspiration from the framework of human rights discourse on North Korean refugees established by Mutua (2001) and refined by Song (2021). It can be understood as the "various integral components or elements of a story and the relationships among these parts ... [including] the character, setting, problem/conflict, plot, and resolution" (Green and McNair, 2019)—that is, a high-level outline which frames a story within a particular political and social context, rather than something which dictates a particular article's linguistic structure. This story grammar structure is useful in analysing the complex and intertwined narratives which the CPC uses in constructing official discourse around COVID-19.

The first component of this story grammar is to conceptualise as a conflict the efforts to prevent and eliminate COVID-19. The CPC consistently employs the metaphor of war in its coverage. The effort to control and prevent the epidemic is a 战斗 [*zhandou*] (battle). Healthcare workers are on the 前线 [*qianxian*] (frontline), while doctors and nurses are characterised as 白衣战士 [*baiyi zhanshi*] (soldiers in white) charging towards 胜利 [*shengli*] (victory). Traditional Chinese idiomatic expressions are combined with bombastic language to paint a vivid image of a collective wartime effort against the enemy of disease, drawing on historical narratives of wartime and revolutionary China to frame an unprecedented public health crisis as a scenario which the Party has successfully overcome before.

The second component is the idolisation of soldiers and healthcare workers within the war on disease as heroes, much like model servicemen of the revolutionary era. The bravery, compassion, and selflessness of these modern-day martyrs on the frontline of public health warfare is underlined by repeated references to the individual sacrifices made for the collective good—not only in terms of risk to physical well-being, but in more abstract sacrifices like separation from loved ones and the mental toll of being on the frontline of a pandemic. These heroes and their sacrifices serve as a model for the populace to emulate through the COVID-19 crisis and reinforce the notion that controlling and eradicating disease is a collective effort, redirecting emotions which might arise out of these crises away from potential criticisms of the Party-State and its handling of the outbreak into an acceptance for the need for selflessness and personal sacrifice.

The final dimension of this story grammar is the characterisation of the CPC as the saviour which will lead China through the COVID-19 crisis to an ultimate victory. The importance of the CPC's leadership in efforts to control COVID-19 is emphasised in every aspect of coverage. Model healthcare heroes are often either already Party members or rewarded with Party membership for their good deeds, integrating their successes in containment and treatment of COVID-19 into the Party's greater efforts.

Here is where the important distinction between "hero" individuals and the "saviour" CPC in COVID-19 discourse lies: while model heroes might be brave and selfless, they will only make a significant contribution to anti-disease efforts acting as a small cog within Party machinery. This approach cements a common understanding of the Communist Party as the paramount authority in China and reaffirms its legitimacy as the continued saviour of the nation.

3. Battle—The Virus as an Enemy: a Timeline of the Militarisation of Anti-Epidemic Efforts

COVID-19 is first mentioned in the *People's Daily* on January 21, 2020, in a policy directive written by Premier Li Keqiang and published on the front page titled "We must put the lives, safety and health of the masses first and resolutely curb the momentum of spread of the epidemic" (Li, 2020, p. 1). January 25 has a handful of articles on the early days of Wuhan's lockdown and efforts to control the spread of the disease. The January 26 front page of the *People's Daily* reads "The epidemic is an order, prevention and control is the responsibility" (*People's Daily*, 2020c, p. 1). From this point on, coverage on the epidemic becomes consistent and efforts to control COVID-19 are regularly couched in terms of warfare.

The battle narrative of COVID-19 (alongside the "hero" and "saviour" aspects of the story grammar) was perfected in a series of three front page on-the-scene reports of the frontline efforts to prevent and control the epidemic in Wuhan, published on February 1, 2, and 5. The three articles are all subtitled "A record from the frontline of defence against the epidemic in Wuhan" and set the standard of battlefield language for all reports to follow—prior to these reports, application of the battle narrative had been inconsistent. The title of the report published on February 2 lays the metaphor out in no uncertain terms: "Hospitals are the battlefield, medical personnel are the soldiers!" (He et al., 2020b, p. 1). This report even reworks content from another report published a week prior to better fit the "battle-hero-saviour" story grammar.

The earlier article published on January 25, 2020 is titled "[We] salute the 'angels in white' going against the current!" (Tian et al., 2020, p. 4) and reports on the bravery and self-sacrifice of healthcare workers on the frontline in Wuhan—here, "going against the current" refers to healthcare workers who did not travel back to their hometowns to celebrate the Chinese New Year with their families, instead remaining in Wuhan to treat patients. While some war imagery is employed (for example, the fight against COVID-19 is referred to as a "battle without gunpowder smoke"), the battle narrative is not particularly heavy-handed, and healthcare workers are mostly framed as ordinary people making sacrifices and working hard to help control the epidemic. The article itself is relatively short and appears on page four of the newspaper.

The front-page report with reworked content published a week later on February 2 has the near identical title "[We] salute the 'soldiers in white' going against the current!" (He at al., 2020c, p. 1). It shares two of the four reporters credited in the article a week prior, it reports on the personal sacrifices made by healthcare workers in Wuhan and includes some of the same content, but its tone is very different. The most obvious change is that healthcare workers are no longer "*angels* in white" but are instead "*soldiers* in white" in the fight against COVID-19. Their colleagues are now 战友 [*zhanyou*] (comrades-in-arms), and the metaphor of a battle is applied throughout. The emotions conveyed by the language used also differ significantly. Compare the closing lines of the two articles:

January 25

During this unusual Chinese New Year's Eve, it is these healthcare workers who bring the warmest and most resolute strength to the country's masses. (Tian et al., 2020, p. 4)

February 2

In Wuhan and across the country, many "soldiers in white" have given up their families for everybody, faced the epidemic and are fighting bravely! They have already resolutely decided: without a complete victory, they pledge not to retreat! We wish the most beautiful "soldiers in white" a safe and triumphant return! (He et al., 2020b, p. 4)

The two other stories in the series are titled "I am a Party member, I will go first!" (He, Li, and Cheng, 2020, p. 1) (February 1) and "First line of defence, stand strong!" (He et al., 2020a, p. 1) (February 5). Together, these three front page reports mark the point where saturation of a hard-line battle narrative and bombastic language reminiscent of revolutionary propaganda becomes the norm in the *People's Daily*'s coverage of the initial COVID-19 outbreak. This sudden, clear, and consistent style change indicates that reporters received direction from above on how to frame their coverage going forward.

The battle narrative continues to feature heavily throughout February and March, with late March seeing the newspaper's first discussions of a return to some sort of normality. The April 7 front page features a picture of Shanxi healthcare workers, who had travelled to Wuhan to assist in efforts, celebrating the end of their post-work quarantine period with the title "Returning home" (*People's Daily*, 2020f, p. 1). The April 8 front page reports on the previous day's announcement that the lockdown in Wuhan would end. From this point on, the *People's Daily* shifts back to more coverage on other issues as the country slowly began to reopen, though regular coverage on COVID-19 continued, albeit with a less prominent battle narrative. As the disorder of COVID-19 began to subside, so too did the need for a stronghold on discourse asserting control over the situation.

3.1 The Implications of a State of War

Framing the effort against COVID-19 as a battle is beneficial to the CPC in several ways. Firstly, it provides the context necessary for the Party to lean on its revolutionary history to position itself as the "saviour" of China during another major crisis, strengthening its legitimacy to rule. Secondly, the metaphor of war justifies to citizens the need for the radical measures undertaken in combat of these diseases—a need to endure short-term hardship to ultimately secure long-term peace and order.

A state of war also invokes an understanding of the need for solidarity and sacrifice for the greater good, which is emphasised in the *People's Daily*. Coverage of COVID-19 frames the pandemic not just as a public health crisis, but as pertaining to the continued success of the 中华民族 [*Zhonghua minzu*] (Chinese nation). Instructions on what must be done to combat the spread of disease lack modifiers like "ideally" or "where possible" and are instead given as an imperative—contrast this with public health instructions from liberal democracies, where stay-at-home orders and mask mandates triggered public debates over government overreach and potential human rights violations (Friedersdorf, 2021; Pew Research Center, 2021; Ore, 2022).

COVID-19 quickly spread on a massive scale and resulted in unprecedented public health controls being taken against hundreds of millions of people. Such a scenario left no room for the *People's Daily* to attempt to minimise the impact on daily life and publish platitudes of cautious optimism, as it did when the SARS epidemic was recognised in 2003; instead, it doubles down on the metaphor of war to maintain a sense of control over the situation. It is worth noting the first mention of Wuhan's COVID-19 outbreak in the *People's Daily* is not accompanied by basic information on the disease, but rather a directive on how it should be combated, illustrating that the publication is not a vehicle for disseminating news but rather serves to propagate the ideology of the Party elite.

4. Hero—The Veneration of Healthcare Workers

Throughout coverage of the initial COVID-19 outbreak, healthcare workers are not only elevated to the status of "soldier" but are venerated alongside members of the People's Liberation Army (PLA) and moulded into models of ideal citizenry resembling the model revolutionary heroes, constructed as near-legendary figures on the public health battlefield. The *People's Daily* acknowledges and utilises the personal suffering and sacrifices of healthcare workers to underline the importance of the work they do in the name of the Party. Discourse around their efforts during the pandemic is constructed to emphasise healthcare workers' place within the greater undertaking of the CPC to achieve victory against the enemy of disease. The sculpting of models is no longer limited to soldiers and healthcare workers; the importance of those who support them—like the delivery drivers who provide supplies, or the construction workers who build new hospitals—is also acknowledged in the *People's Daily*. Healthcare workers, however, are elevated to a level beyond "ordinary" people, and an expectation of their self-sacrifice for the public good is unquestionable.

4.1 Becoming Superhuman

In *People's Daily* coverage, healthcare workers are elevated to an almost "superhuman" status. They are presented as having an undying dedication to their work and a devotion to serving the Chinese people. It is taken for granted that all healthcare workers are self-sacrificing heroes willing to become martyrs for a cause greater than themselves. The article "Salute the 'soldiers in white' going against the current!" published on February 2, 2020 at the height of the lockdown in Wuhan is replete with such sentiments:

> Fever clinic, designated hospital, specialised department, observation zone, isolation zone, "red zone"—these words make ordinary people terrified. However, 60,000 Wuhan medical personnel hold to their posts in the midst of an overwhelming volume of work; more than 15,000 "soldiers in white" are fighting on the front line to control the epidemic. (He et al., 2020b, p. 4)

Here, the white-clad soldiers in the war against disease are explicitly elevated to a status above ordinary citizens.

> In Wuhan and across the country, many "soldiers in white" have given up their families for everybody, faced the epidemic and are fighting bravely! They have already resolutely decided: without a complete victory, they pledge not to retreat! (He et al., 2020b, p. 4)

4.2 Emotions as a Tool

The *People's Daily* assures readers that healthcare workers do not fear hard work or death on the frontline of the war against COVID-19—direct quotes from healthcare workers are scattered across all coverage, assuring readers that "soldiers in white" will stick to their oaths and not burn out or give up in the face of a terrifying and poorly-understood threat. According to the *People's Daily*, the situation is under control and China is being protected by some of its most loyal and steadfast workers.

Notably, there is a layer of humanness and vulnerability in healthcare workers in the discourse of COVID-19 which was absent in model heroes in the revolutionary era—but only to an extent that can be leveraged by the Party. Under Mao Zedong, model heroes did not demonstrate weakness. They were content to unwaveringly carry out their assigned tasks, and did not complain, question orders or express negative or complex emotions.

In *People's Daily* coverage of COVID-19, there is an appeal to human nature. Soldiers in white are depicted as crying from stress, fighting against exhaustion, and expressing a longing for the battle to soon end—but always in a way which does not present as a liability to the epidemic response. There are no mentions in reports of self-doubt about meaning, purpose, or ability—vulnerability in the "model heroes for the epidemic era" tends to focus on guilt about neglecting family to work extended shifts and is framed as a dilemma between competing private and public interests.

The answer to this dilemma in official discourse is always, of course, that the public interest comes first. The Party cannot tolerate compromising its crisis response for the sake of private interests. Nevertheless, the personal sacrifices which healthcare workers make fighting on the frontline of COVID-19 are "made real" in a way which was absent in the revolutionary era.

4.3 The Post-Revolutionary Evolution of Models

The concept of the model is alive and well in COVID-19 discourse, but unlike the revolutionary era the CPC partially acknowledges the humanity of the people they have elevated to "hero" status. The "ideal model" still plays an important part in ideological discourse, but is moulded to circumstance.

Readers of the *People's Daily* are reminded that these healthcare heroes are extraordinary not for performing near-impossible feats, but rather for their steadfastness in the face of danger and disorder and their loyalty to the Party. This echoes a broader shift in official discourse away from the bravery of military serviceman who signed up to serve their country, towards everyday acts of service and heroism by civilians as being central to the nation's welfare in contemporary portrayals of revolutionary-era history heroes (Edwards, 2010, p. 28). Though the *People's Daily* elevates health workers into model heroes, it makes clear that there is no room for individual exceptionalism. These models exist as an example to strive for, but only for personal growth which is for the benefit of society at large.

5. Saviour—The Party Will Undoubtedly Win

Framing public health as battles to be fought and won by soldiers on the frontline, under the leadership of the Party, strengthens the position of the CPC in two ways. Firstly, to frame the fight against COVID as a battle is to understand it as something which can be fought and won. It is not an insurmountable challenge; while the road may be long and difficult, the long revolutionary history of the CPC and its success in previous battles gives confidence that this enemy, too, will eventually be defeated. Understanding COVID-19 in terms of warfare also positions the CPC (a vanguard party with a well-established and repeatedly underlined military history) as the only sensible choice in leading the response, cementing its position as the paramount authority in China. Just as it was the Party which finally brought China out of the Century of Humiliation and through the revolutionary era, only the Party could lead China through the disorder of COVID-19 and into a brighter future.

The CPC as the pillar of China's COVID-19 response is epitomised in the March 26, 2020 editorial "Neither wind nor rain will stop us from forging ahead":

A beacon of strength in a difficult time, standing lofty and tall when the storm hits, calming the great waves. At a critical moment when a country is overcoming difficulties, the stronger its backbone, the more powerful it will be. (Ren, 2020, p. 1)

The editorial details the rapid response to the COVID-19 outbreak "under the strong leadership of the Party Central Committee with Comrade Xi Jinping as the core." The editorial ends with the line: "Wuhan will win! Hubei will win! China will win!" (Ren, 2020, p. 2).

Indeed, the *People's Daily* makes clear that the Party must and will establish and maintain a presence on all frontlines of the epidemic responses. The frontpage of the *People's Daily* on February 1, 2020 reads "since the construction of Leishenshan Hospital began, it is still Party member commandos leading the charge" (He, Li, and Cheng, 2020, p. 1). This reference to the famous makeshift COVID hospital built in only ten days (often used as a symbol of the Party's swift large-scale mobilisation in response to the outbreak) is but one example; similar sentiments can be found in dozens of articles across coverage of COVID-19.

The *People's Daily* also, without publishing any specific complaints, steers discourse away from criticism of the initial handling of the coronavirus outbreak and instead reaffirms the incredible efforts of the CPC. The March 26 editorial also says:

Some people are deeply moved that in the face of an unprecedented epidemic in a country with a population of more than one billion people, water has not stopped, electricity has not stopped, heating has not stopped, communication has not stopped, supply chains have not broken down, and social order has not given way to chaos... Only China, under the leadership of the Communist Party of China, could do this. (Ren, 2020, p. 1)

This serves as a reminder to readers that not only is the CPC doing its utmost to prevent and control the spread of COVID-19, but that they should pause and reflect on the long-term prosperity and social order brought to China by the Communist Party.

Any shortcomings in the CPC's response or non-compliance issues in the wake of mass stay-at-home orders are glossed over; mentions of citizens breaking lockdown rules are few and far between, with only occasional warnings not to become a "deserter" (逃兵 [*taobing*]) and that "[those who] pull away and shirk responsibility must be resolutely held accountable; those who commit dereliction of duty will be investigated and dealt with in accordance with the law" (*People's Daily*, 2020e, p. 1).

Assurances of confidence in the Party's leadership in response to COVID-19 are peppered throughout coverage on the crisis, and often go one step beyond to state outright that there is no alternative to defeating the epidemic but to follow Party orders.

When millions are of one mind, there is no mountain that cannot be climbed; when hearts are joined, there is no hurdle that cannot be crossed. To be confident in winning a victory in the battle against the epidemic, we must unswervingly implement every policy and plan of the Party Central Committee. (*People's Daily*, 2020d, p. 1)

5.1 To be in the Party is Good; to be Good is to be in the Party

The "battle" and "hero" aspects of the story grammar found in the *People's Daily*'s coverage of COVID-19 feed into the "saviour" aspect to reaffirm the legitimacy and moral supremacy of Communist Party rule in China. Healthcare workers are constructed into heroes on the frontline of a battle without gunpowder smoke, and then absorbed by the CPC into the Party machinery to reaffirm the Party's paramount authority.

A February 29 article paraphrasing a speech given by Xi Jinping on February 23 flagged rewarding healthcare workers with Party membership:

It is necessary to promptly publicize and commend Party members, cadres, and exemplary collectives who have performed outstandingly. Party member candidates who have performed outstandingly on the front line of the struggle can join the Party [while still] on the battlefront. (*People's Daily*, 2020b, p. 1)

This hero–Party linkage flows in both directions. Not only are some healthcare workers rewarded with fast-tracked Party membership for their hard work, others apply for Party membership to enhance serving their country on the frontline:

"I volunteer to join the Communist Party of China…" On January 30 Xu Jing, the head nurse of the Intensive Care Unit of Fudan University's Zhongshan Hospital in Shanghai, joined the Party through a remote link while on the battlefront at Wuhan Jinyintan Hospital. She had received the order to set off [to Wuhan] on New Year's Eve and only hurriedly took a few bites of food before picking up her bag. (He et al., 2020b, p. 4)

China's COVID-19 response is fundamentally underpinned by the Party's presence; to be committed to fighting against the public health crisis is to be a good and loyal member of the CPC. Making healthcare workers who fight on the frontline of public health crises into Party members transforms their victories in controlling and preventing the spread of COVID-19 into victories for the Party. Not only does this serve to reassure readers that their faith in the Party to ultimately win this war is well placed, but also reaffirms the CPC's socio-political supremacy and righteousness in ruling China.

6. China Leading the World Against COVID-19

In the *People's Daily*, the disruption of COVID-19 is merely one battlefront of a greater global war as China challenges American hegemony and leads the global fight against COVID-19. In the early days of the COVID-19 outbreak (when the virus was generally viewed as a China-centric issue), *People's Daily* coverage on the international response to the Wuhan outbreak emphasised the strength of CPC leadership and the confidence the international community had in China's response.

As COVID-19 came under control in China but exploded globally, coverage shifted towards a narrative of China stepping up to aid other countries. Indeed, the March 30, 2020 article "Helping the whole world fight the pandemic demonstrates the responsibilities of a major power (an expert explains)" not only affirms the CPC's self-perception of China as having graduated to "major power" status, but lays out clearly its intent to act as a sensible international leader.

> "If you want to go fast, go alone; if you want to go far, go together." China has always advocated building a "community with a shared future for mankind," upholding and safeguarding multilateralism, upholding openness, cooperation, and win-win ideals, and actively participating in and resolving the shared problems faced by the international community. China, acting in the role of an open, cooperative, and leading major power in the international community, is a reliable partner in the international family. In the future, China will continue to build consensus, unite partners, and provide assistance within the scope of its capabilities. (Liu, 2020, p. 10)

As international tensions rose in the face of COVID-19, the pro-democracy movement in Hong Kong and increased attention towards the treatment of the Uyghur ethnic group in Xinjiang, the *People's Daily* also became very direct in its criticism of the US. From May 1 to May 7, 2020, the newspaper published seven daily editorials in the series "Spreading rumours and slander about China's anti-epidemic efforts runs contrary to international justice" (Zhong, 2020e, p. 3) under the pseudonym *Zhong Sheng* (a homonym for 中声 [*Zhongsheng*], literally "voice of China").

The articles defend and extol China's efforts in controlling the global spread of COVID-19 through the provision of aid and expertise, hit back against accusations of China underreporting domestic COVID-19 case numbers, and take an extremely strong position against American politicians who have criticised China. They accuse American politicians and news outlets of being liars and hypocrites, declaring that they only defame China to draw attention away from the US's 灾难性 [*zainanxing*] (catastrophic) response to the COVID-19 pandemic (Zhong, 2020b).

The editorial on May 3, 2020 calls out American leadership's flip-flopping between praising and criticising China's COVID-19 response, while also stating that the origins of COVID-19 as Chinese have not been definitively proven and suggesting that the US itself is hiding information on the origins of COVID-19 outbreaks (Zhong, 2020a); the May 4 and 6 editorials titled "How can you talk of human rights when you ignore the sanctity of life?" (Zhong, 2020c) and "Prattling on about 'loving others as you love yourself,' but in actuality [you are] selfish and cold-blooded" (Zhong, 2020d) highlight the contradiction between the US's alleged status as a proponent of human rights in the face of thousands of US citizens dying with COVID-19 every day. This particular framing of the US government and media as hypocritical liars would continue on into coverage and criticism of the US's position on the 2020 Hong Kong protests as the year progressed.

The lengthy two-page spread "America's lies concerning China about the novel coronavirus pneumonia epidemic, and the real truth" published May 10, 2020 directly addresses and rebuts twenty-four "lies", including "The virus was caused by Chinese people eating bats" and "China's political system is the source of the problem" (*People's Daily*, 2020a, pp. 3–4). The article weaves arguments against what it calls racist misconceptions alongside discussions of the CPC's strength, openness, and cooperation with the international community, and anger towards what it perceives as deceitful and hypocritical criticism levelled by the US towards China.

The *People's Daily*'s coverage of the domestic and international response to COVID-19 characterises the Chinese government as a responsible, powerful, and cooperative international leader which will not be hampered by the efforts of international rivals who would sacrifice the well-being of both their own citizens and the broader global community in an ill-fated attempt to stifle China's continuing rise.

There is also a marked emphasis not just on the importance of Party leadership, but on Xi Jinping being the core of the Party. Directions on controlling and preventing the spread of the outbreak are not just given by the Party, but the Party *under the leadership of Xi Jinping*. Repeated reference is made to Xi 亲自 [*qinzi*] (personally) issuing commands and deploying people and resources. This emphasis on the General Secretary's role in the Party is a marked difference from the comparatively infrequent references to Hu Jintao (then General Secretary) in the *People's Daily* during the SARS epidemic, and reflects the broader centralisation of power and CPC leadership in the Xi Jinping era.

7. Conclusion

By framing the disruption of COVID-19 as a war and frontline workers as heroic soldiers fighting on the battlefield of disease, the Communist Party of China seeks to shape discourse around COVID-19 to position itself as the only entity which can lead the country through the public health crisis, thereby strengthening its political legitimacy. The *People's Daily* has a clear pattern of how it communicates the CPC's role in COVID-19, and the integration of frontline healthcare workers into the Party is reflective of the emphasis on unification between the Party-State and the masses in broader Chinese government discourse. As the CPC sees it, the Party should play a leading role not just when responding to the threat of disease, but in all aspects of the lives of Chinese people.

In an era marked by China's emerging global superpower status and the absence of any hesitancy in confronting countries which might seek to block its rise, an understanding of how the CPC perceives itself and its role in both domestic and international governance has never been more relevant. Shaping discourse to emphasise the importance of the CPC in China's continued success, and the importance of China's leadership in the international response to major crises like COVID-19, leaves the Party in a stronger position for possible crises in the future which might otherwise pose a serious threat to its rule.

Though this chapter has focused on the initial 2020 outbreak, new rounds of outbreaks, lockdowns, and protests in China in 2022 have posed even greater challenges to the CPC, as well as a revival of the *People's Daily*'s "battle-hero-saviour" story grammar. Nevertheless, the CPC is unafraid to point out the hundreds of thousands of COVID-19 deaths in major Western democracies as proof of the failings of these countries, continuing a pattern of rejecting the "Western model" of government and governance which has accompanied the rise of Xi Jinping and the erosion of pluralisation of decision-making at the highest levels of Chinese politics. No longer is China content to simply "engage" in international diplomacy; the COVID-19 pandemic has given the CPC another opportunity to challenge American hegemony and assert China's role as an international leader.

Susanna Ackroyd is a policy analyst working in Melbourne, Australia. She holds First Class Honours from the Asia Institute, University of Melbourne. She also holds a Bachelor of Asia-Pacific Studies in Chinese language and Asia-Pacific politics from the Australian National University.

References

Bakken, Børge. 2000. *The Exemplary Society: Human Improvement, Social Control, and the Dangers of Modernity in China*. New York: Oxford University Press.

Edwards, Louise. 2010. "Military celebrity in China: The evolution of 'Heroic and Model Servicemen.'" In *Celebrity in China*, edited by Louise Edwards and Elaine Jeffreys, 21–43. Hong Kong: Hong Kong University Press.

Friedersdorf, Conor. 2021. "Australia traded away too much liberty." *The Atlantic*, September 2, 2021. https://www.theatlantic.com/ideas/archive/2021/09/pandemic-australia-still-liberal-democracy/619940/.

Green, Marybeth, and C. Lisa McNair. 2019. "Steamsational writing: An investigation into using robots to inspire children's narrative skills." In *Handbook of Research on Integrating Digital Technology With Literacy Pedagogies*, edited by Pamela M. Sullivan, Jessica L. Lantz and Brian A. Sullivan, 175–191. Hershey: IGI Global.

Gries, Peter Hays. 2007. "Narratives to live by: The century of humiliation and Chinese national identity today." In *China's Transformations: The Stories Beyond the Headlines*, edited by Lionel M. Jensen and Timothy B. Weston, 112–127. Lanham: Rowman & Littlefield.

He, Guanghua, Changyu Li, and Yuanzhou Cheng. 2020. "Wo shi dangyuan, wo xian shang!" [I am a Party member, I will go first!]. *People's Daily*, February 1.

He, Guanghua, Changyu Li, Yuanzhou Cheng, and Haotian Fan. 2020a. "Di-yi dao fangxian, shouzhu!" [First line of defence, stand strong!]. *People's Daily*, February 5.

He, Guanghua, Doudou Tian, Yuanzhou Cheng, and Shaotie Shen. 2020b. "Zhijing! Nixing de "baiyi zhanshi!" [We salute the 'soldiers in white' going against the current!]. *People's Daily*, February 2, 2020.

Jeffreys, Elaine, and Xuezhong Su. 2016. "Governing through Lei Feng: A Mao-era role model in reform-era China." In *New Mentalities of Government in China*, edited by David Bray and Elaine Jeffreys, 30–55. Abingdon: Routledge.

Li, Keqiang. 2020. "Yao ba renmin qunzhong shengming anquan he shenti jiankang fang zai di-yi wei jianjue ezhi yiqing manyan shitou" [We must put the lives, safety and health of the masses first and resolutely curb the momentum of spread of the epidemic]. *People's Daily*, January 21, 2020.

Liu, Xiao. 2020. "Yuanzhu quanqiu zhan 'yi' zhangxian daguo dandang (zhuanjia jiedu)" [Helping the whole world fight the pandemic demonstrates the responsibilities of a major power (an expert explains)]. *People's Daily*, March 30, 2020.

Ore, Adeshola. 2022. "Rights watchdog sees 1,445% spike in questions about Victorian government's powers during Covid." *The Guardian*, March 23, 2022. https://www.theguardian.com/australia-news/2022/mar/23/rights-watchdog-sees-1445-spike-in-questions-about-victorian-governments-powers-during-covid.

People's Daily. 2020a. "Meiguo guanyu xinguan feiyan yiqing de she Hua huangyan yu shishi zhenxiang" [America's lies concerning China about the novel coronavirus pneumonia epidemic, and the real truth]. May 10, 2020.

People's Daily. 2020b. "Chongfen fahui dangyuan ganbu xianfeng mofan zuoyong" [Bring into full play Party members' and cadres' pioneering and exemplary roles]. February 29, 2020.

People's Daily. 2020c. "Yiqing jiushi mingling Fangkong jiushi zeren" [The epidemic is an order, prevention and control is the responsibility]. January 26, 2020.

People's Daily. 2020d. "Jianding xinxin jianjue da ying yiqing fangkong zuji zhan" [Have steadfast confidence in resolutely winning the fight to prevent and control the epidemic]. January 26, 2020.

People's Daily. 2020e. "Wei daying yiqing fangkong zujizhan tigong youli baozhang" [Provide a strong guarantee to win the epidemic prevention and control blockade]. February 17, 2020.

People's Daily. 2020f. "Huijia" [Returning home]. April 7, 2020.

People's Daily Online. n.d. "Introduction to People's Daily." Accessed May 21, 2021. http://en.people.cn/90827/90828/index.html.

Pew Research Center. 2021. "A year of U.S. public opinion on the coronavirus pandemic." March 5, 2023. https://www.pewresearch.org/2021/03/05/a-year-of-u-s-public-opinion-on-the-coronavirus-pandemic/.

Ren, Zhongping. 2020. "Fengyu wuzu xiang qian jin" [Neither wind nor rain will stop us from forging ahead]. *People's Daily*, March 26, 2020.

Song, Jay. 2021. "The 'Savage–Victim–Saviour' story grammar of the North Korean human rights industry." *Asian Studies Review* 45, no. 1: 48–66.

Tian, Doudou, Yuanzhou Cheng, Haotian Fan, and Jun Wu. 2020. "Zhijing! Nixiang er xing de baiyi tianshi" [We salute the 'angels in white' going against the current!]. *People's Daily*, January 25, 2020.

Wang, Haiyang, Colin Sparks, and Yu Huang. 2018. "Measuring differences in the Chinese press: A study of People's Daily and Southern Metropolitan Daily." *Global Media and China* 3, no. 3: 125–140.

Zhao, Suisheng. 1998. "A state-led nationalism: The patriotic education campaign in Post-Tiananmen China." *Communist and Post-Communist Studies* 31, no. 3: 287–302.

Zhong, Sheng. 2020a. "Zhui ze suopei naoju shi wenming zhi chi" [Farcically claiming damages is a disgrace to civility]. *People's Daily*, May 3, 2020.

Zhong, Sheng. 2020b. "'Shuai guo' qineng zhengjiu shengming" [How could 'passing the buck' save lives?]. *People's Daily*, May 2.

Zhong, Sheng. 2020c. "Moshi 'shengming zhishang' he tan renquan" [How can you talk of human rights when you ignore the 'sanctity of life'?]. *People's Daily*, May 4, 2020.

Zhong, Sheng. 2020d. "Konghan 'airen ru ji' shize zisi lengxue" [Prattling on about 'loving others as you love yourself,' but in actuality selfish and cold-blooded]. *People's Daily*, May 6, 2020.

Zhong, Sheng. 2020e. "Wuming hua shi weixian de 'zhengzhi bingdu'" [Stigmatisation is a dangerous "political virus"]. *People's Daily*, May 1, 2020.

CHAPTER 3

What Has Machine Translation "Mis-Translated" about COVID-19? What "Mistakes" Can Tell Us about Humanity that Machines Cannot

Wayne Wen-chun Liang, Ester S.M. Leung & Chun Hin Tse

Abstract

This chapter examines the performance of a Neural Machine Translation (NMT) model in the translations of Chinese language journal articles on COVID-19. The limitations of existing automatic evaluation metrics for translation quality are identified, and both House's (2015) refined translation quality assessment model and the Multidimensional Quality Metric model (Lommel et al., 2014) are applied to identify semantic and pragmatic errors. The authors argue that automatic evaluation metrics would benefit from the introduction of cultural, emotional, or ideological elements as these are necessary to understand the discursive, pragmatic, and social communication rendered by humans. Rather than relying solely on automatic evaluation metrics, a consolidated model of human-intervened evaluation should be applied to pinpoint specific translation problems produced by machine translation.

Keywords: Neural Machine Translation, automatic evaluation metrics, Juliane House's translation quality assessment model, multidimensional quality metric model, machine translation

1. Introduction

For some time, human beings have used computers to carry out fully or partially automatic processes to translate texts from one language to another. Machine translation (MT) has evolved through different phases since the 1950s from rule- and dictionary-based approaches through to the statistical approach and, finally, to the neural-network-based approach. Whereas the early development of MT endeavoured to mimic human cognition, advancements in machine learning and data science have moved the later development of MT gradually towards mass industrial translation.

Shaken by the outbreak of COVID-19 in late 2019, demands for information have grown exponentially. One of the most significant endeavours of healthcare practitioners, scientists, and researchers in combating this global pandemic is the sharing of information. Faced with the threat of illness and the disruption of our daily lives, we all endeavour to seek remedies, be they medical, social, or economic. Making information accessible across different cultural contexts is essential, as it could constitute an effective approach to fighting COVID-19 and its second- and third-order effects.

During the COVID-19 pandemic, scientific papers and preprints in various research areas, such as epidemiology, biomedical engineering, environmental science, and socioeconomics flooded into academic venues to flesh out our understanding of coronavirus. This could also be seen from the World Health Organization's (WHO) website, which has constantly been publishing COVID-related information (see https://search.bvsalud.org/global-literature-on-novel-coronavirus-2019-ncov/). As of July 21, 2021, a total of 310,813 scientific findings have been published on WHO's COVID-19 database; amongst them, 1,174 are scientific papers written in English, sharing information about COVID-19 from the perspective of traditional Chinese medicine (TCM). However, most Chinese-language articles about applying TCM in the diagnosis and treatment of COVID-19 have not been translated into other languages and so are still not widely available in other parts of the world. This could result in a vacuum of information sharing about COVID-19 written in Chinese. Using MT to tackle this problem could facilitate the transmission of knowledge, but the quality of MT, especially in the areas in which it underperforms, such as the low-resource domains, is still uncertain and further investigation is needed.

Machine learning technology simulates how neurons work in human brains whereby an "interconnected web of neurons transmitting elaborate patterns of electrical signals" and "dendrites receive input signals and, based on those inputs, fire an output signal via an axon" (Shiffman, 2012, p. 466). The neural network is understood as a nexus of systems which can access and process information from multiple directions simultaneously, rather than linearly or procedurally. The new state of the art in MT—Neural Machine Translation (NMT)—is modelled on the principle that statistical data are retrieved and processed for recognised patterns rather than for individual grammatical items. NMT has indeed achieved state-of-the-art results in most situations.

For NMT, the availability of large and high-quality datasets is of great importance (Dunder, Seljan, and Pavlovski, 2020, p. 1278). In other words, a good NMT requires a huge amount of data to train a model to attain good translation performance. However, an MT system is unlikely to achieve high performance in a new domain where there is little or no labelled data. As Jin et al. (2020) state, NMT systems are data-hungry and would normally perform poorly in new domains where resources are scarce. The accuracy of NMT is therefore often questioned, as MT may perform poorly in emerging domains on current topical issues with no parallel data, for example, the COVID-19 pandemic in relation to laws, medicine, and technology. Similarly, an NMT model would not be able to achieve satisfactory results in low-resourced languages, as datasets for less-spoken languages would be in short supply, as shown in Dunder et al.'s (2020) study.

The acquisition and preparation of datasets, however, is often labour intensive and time consuming. First of all, the relevant data need to be crawled and examined to ensure quality; then, the data must be input into selected programs. In order to overcome the problem of scarcity of parallel datasets, a domain adaptation approach has been considered. In general, domain adaptation for MT has three scenarios: supervised, unsupervised, and semi-supervised (Jin et al., 2020). In the supervised domain adaptation setting, both the source and target domains have parallel data; in the unsupervised domain adaptation setting, neither the source nor the target domain has parallel data; and in the semi-supervised domain adaptation setting, only the source domain has parallel data, and the target domain does not.

Based on the domain adaption model, this chapter aims to (1) examine how the NMT model performs in a low-resource domain, such as the COVID-19-related texts; (2) identify the areas in which the MT evaluation metrics fail to reflect the quality of translation; and (3) explore the tendency of common errors made by the NMT model.

Recent studies concerning the accuracy and efficiency of MT have been conducted to compare several MT systems with the same test set (see, for example, Amancio et al. [2011]). Other studies have examined the automatic quality assessment metrics on MT in various domains (i.e., Seljan and Dunder, 2015a) and have analysed and compared the quality of the MT systems between automatic and human evaluations (i.e., Seljan and Dunder, 2015b; Seljan, Tucaković, and Dunder, 2015).

An automatic MT quality evaluation can be performed using the following common metrics: BiLingual Evaluation Understudy (BLEU), National Institute of Standards and Technology (NIST), Metric for Evaluation of Translation with Explicit ORdering (METEOR) and General Text Matcher (GTM) (Seljan and Dunder, 2015a). Amongst the four metrics, BLEU has become almost a de facto automatic evaluation method for assessing the quality of an MT system. BLEU is a metric which scores the similarity between two texts. This would involve an evaluation between the machine-produced translation and the referenced human-produced translation (often referred to as the gold standard). According to Dunder et al. (2020, p. 1281), "BLEU matches machine-translated n-grams with n-grams of its reference translation, and counts the numbers of matches, most often for 1–4 n-grams." This means that the BLEU score is based on the degree of overlapping words between the two translations at the sentence level; therefore, it is not indexical of the accuracy of the translation. The BLEU score drops when the machine-translated and reference n-grams match less frequently over larger ranges. The metric score of BLEU can range from zero, that is, none of the words in the machine-translated and reference translation match, to one, that is, a complete overlap of the machine-translated and reference translation (ibid.). Generally speaking, if the BLEU of a machine-translated target text is above 0.3 (30), the MT version is considered understandable, whereas if the BLEU of a machine-translated target text is above 0.5 (50), the translation is regarded as fluent and good.

2. Method

2.1 Preparation and Pre-processing of the Data

An NMT model typically requires a huge amount of high-quality data to train it, so the preparation and pre-processing phases are fundamental to this project. A standard NMT model uses bilingual parallel corpora (also known as bitext) as the training data, consisting of sentence pairs of the concerned languages deemed parallel to one another. Ordinarily, NMT does not take translation direction into consideration; that is, either English or Chinese could be the source language or target language. Hence, a source sentence and its target translation in any direction would be considered parallel. Two sentences coproduced in different languages would also be considered parallel to each other.

However, when dealing with texts from a specific domain, such as medical, legal, or scientific, the language and terms might vary widely, and some common words might have different meanings in a specific domain. For example, the word "consideration" in a legal contract could mean the amount of money paid for a property, whereas in a general context it means the act of thinking carefully about something. It is ideal if parallel data of the specific domain are available as training data, but this is rarely the case. More often, parallel data are extremely scarce for certain specific domains, as is the case with bitexts about COVID-19. When the global pandemic emerged in late 2019, texts about COVID-19 were mostly written in English and large, high-quality bilingual datasets in this domain remain scarce—these are considered to be low-resource data for training purposes. To tackle low-resource settings in a specific domain, researchers have proposed *domain adaptation*, which involves using generic bilingual data as its base and domain-specific data for fine tuning. Domain adaptation involves leveraging abundant generic parallel data to assist with training the NMT model in low-resource domains. The standard domain adaptation problem assumes a large generic bilingual parallel dataset, coupled with a much smaller bilingual domain-specific parallel dataset, whereas semi-supervised domain adaptation assumes the same large generic bilingual parallel dataset, but with non-parallel domain-specific data.

2.1.1 Model Architecture

In this study, we adopted the standard transformer encoder–decoder, with shared sub-word vocabulary as our architecture. We pretrained parameters from monolingual texts, with which we initialised the encoder and decoder of our model. The standard transformer, proposed by Vaswani et al. (2018), is the most prevalent architecture used in NMT. We made the architectural decision based on Jin et al. (2020), as they focused on tackling a semi-supervised domain adaptation problem which is similar to the problem we faced in this study.

2.1.2 Training Method

We have no access to the domain-specific data in one of the languages involved in translation. Therefore, differing from Jin et al.'s (2020) research, which assumes the provision of parallel generic bilingual data and non-parallel domain-specific data, we selected a one-time back-translation approach (Sennrich, Haddow, and Birch, 2016), a widely adopted method which has been shown to be competitive compared with other baselines in most data settings. This approach involves first training a generic NMT model using out-domain parallel data and then using the trained model to translate monolingual domain-specific data into the other language to produce a pseudo-parallel corpus. These pseudo-parallel data from the original domain-specific sentences and the machine-translated sentences are then used to train the domain-specific NMT model. As pretraining was shown to improve NMT performance in Lample and Conneau's work (2019) and was also adopted in domain adaptation by Jin et al. (2020), we initialised both models with the pretrained parameters described in the model architecture.

2.1.3 Datasets

We have adopted the COVID-19 domain-specific datasets written in English and Chinese and collected a total of four datasets in our experiment. For pretraining, we used the English and Chinese texts from the Wikipedia dump (https://dumps. wikimedia.org), an open-access dataset which consists of a large number of articles from Wikipedia and covers a wide range of domains. It was also used as the pretraining data in both Lample and Conneau's (2019) and Jin et al.'s (2020) studies. To train the generic model, we used the AI Challenger 2018 dataset, a high-quality industry sample dataset released by Sogo. We selected the CORD-19 dataset (https://www.kaggle.com/allen-institute-for-ai/CORD-19-research-challenge) as our target domain-specific monolingual data. This dataset consists of large volumes of government, news, and academic English texts which concern COVID-19. We extracted all body texts from the raw XML data and further removed all texts which had empty or non-English titles. Finally, we filtered the remaining texts to prune any non-English sentences, resulting in a monolingual corpus of 5,154,062 English sentences in the COVID-19 domain.

For validation and evaluation, we obtained COVID-19-related articles from the CNKI Journal Translation Project. In total, we collected 121 open-access paragraph-aligned articles via web crawling. We used two sentence boundary detection tools (i.e., PySBD for English and TR4W for Chinese) to break the English and Chinese paragraphs into sentences. We then selected paragraphs which yielded an identical number of sentences, from which we gathered 2,381 sentence pairs via manual alignment. The remaining sentences were encoded using a pretrained encoder from LASER (https://github.com/facebookresearch/LASER), and the cosine distance of the encoded representations of the sentence pairs was measured. In all, 639 of them had a similarity higher than 0.9 (on a scale of 0 to 1, with "1" denoting an identical match). These likely aligned sentence pairs were extracted from the CNKI Journal Translation Project and appended to the first 976 of the manually aligned sentences as validation data. The remaining 1,405 manually aligned sentence pairs were reserved for manual evaluation.

2.2 Translation Quality Assessment: The Housian Approach

In an attempt to bridge the gap between computer-assessed and human-assessed translation output, we sought to augment the evaluation metrics of BLEU of MT based on House's (1997) model. The evaluation of BLEU is position-independent, meaning the analysis is based on the sequences of consecutive words at the sentence level without considering the context of the text. For example, the two sentences—"I am sick" and "Sick, I am"—would receive almost the same BLEU scores except for the bigram measurement of the n-grams "am sick" and "Sick I am." On the other hand, when human assessors examine the quality of a translation, they consider not only the linguistic coherence of the translation to the original text, but also the extralinguistic aspects, such as functionality, rhetoric, and the emotional factors of the translation.

There is never an easy answer to the simple question: Is this a good translation? Papineni et al. (2002) claim that BLEU is a reliable MT evaluation metric since it correlates with human evaluation for individual sentence judgment, but translation is never simply an act of rendering one language into another; it is preconditioned by the languages and cultures in which the communication is based (Gentzler, 2017). The evaluation carried out by BLEU is only a score of the matched n-grams between the reference translation and the MT version. Readability and acceptability of a translation, depending on whether the target text is equivalent to the source text at the semantic level as well as at the pragmatic level, cannot be assessed through BLEU. Bassnett (2003, p. 4) argues that "the translator is ... a creative artist who ensures the survival of writing across time and space, an intercultural mediator and interpreter, a figure whose importance to the continuity and diffusion of culture is immeasurable." If the process of translation also encompasses making cultural otherness comprehensible to target readers, we would have to reconsider whether BLEU can sufficiently reflect the actual quality of the MT version.

Evaluating MT quality has become increasingly important, especially for industrialised MT output. For human evaluation, a common approach is to employ bilingual translators to assess the MT output based on the accuracy of lexical meanings (such as preserving the original meaning of the source text in the target text) and language rules (by the appropriate use of the target syntactic structure) (Popović, 2018). Very often, a five-point scale is used to evaluate whether the output is equivalent to the source text on a sentence basis. Such an approach, however, confines the examination of translation quality to "a comparison of the two texts and the resultant assessment of their relative match" (House, 2009, p. 224). The readability of a translation is imperative when transferring knowledge, especially when disseminating updated scientific information about fighting a global pandemic such as COVID-19.

Regarding the human assessment of translation quality, House's translation quality assessment (TQA) model (1977/1981) is an early attempt to use pragmatic theories to analyse the language in use as well as the situational–cultural particularities of the source and target texts. House's model is based on the concept of equivalence: an evaluation must go beyond "formal, syntactic and lexical similarities ... because any two linguistic items in two different languages are multiply ambiguous, and because languages cut up reality in different ways" (House, 2001, p. 247). For House (1997), the equivalence of meaning lies in three aspects: semantic, pragmatic, and textual, which considers the equivalence of meaning to be more than just the relations between verbal signs in the source and target languages. It is also the correlation between the verbal signs and how they are used in a communicative situation. Saldanha and O'Brien (2014) highlight the following three aspects of the evaluation of translation quality: the process of translation, the context of translation, and the product itself. Hence, a translation should be considered "the recontextualization of a text in L1 by a semantically and pragmatically equivalent text in L2," and the evaluation of translation quality should take into consideration not only semantic equivalence, but also pragmatic equivalence (House, 2001, p. 247).

House's refined TQA model (1997) further addresses the interdependency of language, situation, and culture in the assessment of translation quality. The model follows the Hallidayan systemic functional theory to select and classify texts for analysis, particularly based on the aspects of register, genre, and language/text. While register deals with the context of a situation for the appropriate use of language, genre is considered to be a cultural discourse consisting of different lexical and grammatical units belonging to their respective cultural discourses. In other words, genre is used to determine cultural discourses, while register defines how and of what the context is made.

On the basis of textual function, as well as the linguistic features and social function of a text, House (1977/1981, p. 49) emphasises that "the function of a text … can be determined by 'opening up' the linguistic materials in terms of the … set of extralinguistic, situational constraints." House's revised TQA model takes into account the interactions between text and context through an inextricable connection between the social environment and the functional organisation of language.

Given that House's (1997) refined model is the most comprehensive model of translation quality assessment in the field of translation studies, this study explores how this model could be used to craft a metric for the human evaluation of MT. However, we recognise a limitation of House's model: its generalisation of error taxonomies, especially for analysis at the sentence level. Hence, we also adopt Lommel et al.'s (2014) flexible Multidimensional Quality Metric (MQM) model to annotate error categories from the MT output during the human assessment process to better understand the errors from the semantic and pragmatic perspectives, and ensure that the human analysis is objective and reliable. MQM categorises errors into two aspects—accuracy and fluency—each containing relevant sub-aspects specific to the issue. In terms of accuracy, the errors include Terminology, Mistranslation, Omission, Addition, and Untranslated, while in terms of fluency, the errors include Style, Spelling, Grammar, Typography, and Unintelligible (Lommel et al., 2014).

3. Errors in Translating COVID-19

As described previously, we assumed a semi-supervised domain adaptation setting in which we had access to abundant parallel generic data and monolingual target domain data. We used back translation, adopting shared vocabulary and applying the standard transformer from Jin et al.'s (2020) work. In Hassan et al. (2018), the authors report that the MT output achieved human parity, with a BLEU score greater than 28 on the context-free sentence translation. The machine output scored 22.3 in BLEU in our experiment, indicating a sub-optimal, yet understandable, product from the MT. Nevertheless, the BLEU score only offers a reference point for how well the NMT model performed generally, without providing specific translation errors. Based only on this score, the MT output is clearly distinguishable from human translations, yet the specific errors or types of errors are still unknown without a human-intervened evaluation.

The human-intervened evaluation in this study is based on a quality assessment of translations from 1,405 manually aligned sentence pairs, extracted from the 121 open-access paragraph-aligned TCM- and COVID-19-related articles collected from the CNKI Journal Translation Project. We used House's model (1997) as an overarching framework and supplemented it with Lommel et al.'s (2014) guidelines regarding MQM for error annotation. The results show that a total of 803 errors in seven sub-categories were produced by the trained NMT model (see Appendix 1).

According to Lommel et al. (2014), if a sentence contains multiple errors at the same level in the hierarchy, only one error type should be counted, and the error which appears first should be selected. For example, the sentence 1.4 麻黄-苍术治疗新冠肺炎的潜在靶点预测 [*1.4 ma huang-cang zhu zhi liao xin guan fei yan de qian zai ba dian yu ce*] (1.4 prediction of potential targets for the treatment of new coronavirus) contains two errors, but the omission of 麻黄-苍术 [*ma huang-cang zhu*] appears first, so the error was annotated as an omission. In total, 692 of the 803 identified errors concerned accuracy, which correlates with the low BLEU score achieved in the automatic evaluation. Mistranslation was the most frequent error type, with 408 occurrences, mainly resulting from the NMT model mistranslating lexical meanings, classical Chinese fixed/idiomatic expressions and TCM-related concepts. Terminology was the second most frequent error type, with 265 instances. See Appendix 1 for the number of errors and some extracted examples.

4. Discussion: What Do the "Errors" Say about MT?

Reiss (1989) explains that the dimensions of language use in an informative text involve transmitting information logically and clearly; presumably, such transmission also reveals the idiosyncrasies of language use in the evaluation text we adopted, given that they are journal articles concerning TCM and COVID-19. At the linguistic level, the language function of such a text type consists of referential or conceptual values, and the level of formality of the language is high, often "well structured, elaborate, logically sequenced, and strongly cohesive" (House, 1977/1981, pp. 41–42), so as to clearly transmit knowledge to readers.

Translating TCM texts is known to be difficult, not only because of the ingredients or herbs which are used, but also because of the different ways in which the body and sickness itself are conceptualised and represented linguistically. A fundamental concept such as 气 [*qi*] (air), which involves not just the lung as an organ, but also the circulation of blood as an energy flow throughout the body, has usually been rendered as "qi" in previous translations, rather than "air" or "gas" as in the MT version. The processes by which a Chinese medicine doctor diagnoses the cause(s) of a health problem, which are called 望 [*wang*] (look) (meaning: checking by sight), 闻 [*wen*] (listen) (checking by listening), 问 [*wen*] (ask) (checking by asking) and 切 [*qie*] (analyse) (analysing the different factors observed), were rendered by the MT as "hope," "smell," "ask," and "cut." It could be inferred that the insufficient number of TCM datasets limited the NMT model's capacity to produce the more domain-specific vocabulary.

Another example can be seen in the segment 从临床表现来看, 新冠肺炎患者重型, 危重型患者病程中可为中, 低热, 甚至无明显发热 [*cong lin chuang biao xian lai kan, xin guan fei yan huan zhe zhong xing, wei zhong xing huan zhe bing cheng zhong ke wei zhong, di re, shen zhi wu ming xian fa re*] and its MT version: "in terms of clinical manifestations, severe, low-grade fever in patients with new coronavirus-induced pneumonia and even no significant fever." We can assume that the Chinese phrase 表现 [*biao xian*] was translated to "manifestations" as a result of the generic dataset used in the training process, as it is not a common word used in the medical field in English. The errors in the sub-category of Mistranslation are thus to be expected, because the datasets in our experiment were mainly composed of COVID-19-domain-specific research reports and academic journals.

Terminology was the second most frequent error type in the human assessment, particularly terminologies for the Chinese medicine ingredients, such as 红参 [*hong shen*] (red ginseng), which was mistranslated as "pork ginseng," and 杏仁 [*xing ren*] (almond nuts), mistranslated as "peanut." Technologically speaking, this kind of problem can be easily solved with better input data, such as a more accurate, parallel bilingual dataset and the use of established glossaries relevant to the texts, but domain-specific, computer-accessible texts on topics such as TCM and COVID-19 are rare, and data preparation requires significant effort.

Some of the mistranslated terminologies involve more complicated processing issues regarding concepts and cognitive perceptions related to the body and to the different systems of medicine. In fact, when comparing the errors the NMT model made in translating terminology, we found that errors related to TCM terms were distinctly more common than those related to COVID-19 terms. This is somewhat expected, however, as only COVID-19-related data were provided as target domain-specific data during training, and the TCM-related data were missing.

Regarding the errors in the aspect of fluency, the most common sub-category identified in the MT was Grammar (58 occurrences). Since the source text is an academic, scientific journal publication, a detailed description of the facts and timeline is crucial for an accurate understanding of the causes, effects, and consequences of events as they happened. In the segment 死亡比率下降除与医疗资源显著改善相关外, 适当的抗病毒治疗和中医药物使用,也可能发挥了一定作用 [*si wang bi lü xia jiang chu yu yi liao zi yuan xian zhu gai shan xiang guan wai, shi dang de kang bing du zhi liao he zhong yi yao wu shi yong, ye ke neng fa hui le yi ding zuo yong*], the Chinese original was translated into "the decrease in the death ratio, in addition to its correlation with significant improvement in medical resources, appropriate antiviral therapy and the use of traditional Chinese medicine may also play a role." Rather than present tense ("may play a role"), use of perfect aspect ("may also have played a role") would have helped to indicate something which had happened in the past. Another example can be seen in the segment 据世界卫生组织(WHO)不完全统计,人 类历史上曾爆发了天花、黑死病(学名"鼠疫") ...等10大传染病疫情扩散事件 [*ju shi jie wei sheng zu zhi (WHO) bu wan quan tong ji, ren lei li shi shang ceng bao fa le tian hua, hei si bing (xue ming "shu yi") ... deng 10 da chuan ran bing yi qing kuo san shi jian*] and its MT version "according to the *world health organization (who)*, human history has been a major outbreak of smallpox, black death (known as "plague") ... and poliomyelitis (also known as "polio")." The incomplete presentative construction ("has been" instead of "there has been") and the use of singular forms to refer several different outbreaks are considered errors in the sub-category of Grammar. The correct form would be "in human history, there have been major outbreaks."

In seeking to correlate the errors annotated from the MQM model with House's TQA model, we will discuss correlations in the following dimensions of language use in terms of field, tenor and mode based on House's model (2015, p. 28):

1. Medium: simple/complex
2. Participation: simple/complex
3. Social role relationship
4. Social attitude
5. Province

House (2015) distinguishes different types of writing and argues that writing which is intended to be spoken as if it were not written would be a manifestation of a complex medium because there is a "specific manner of text constitution, particular theme-rheme sequencing, subjectivity ... and high redundancy" (ibid., p. 28), while a text written to be read would be of a simple medium. As for Participation, a text would have simple participation if it were a monologue or dialogue, but would be complex if the monologue involved various forms of indirect participation, elicitation, or indirect addresses. Since the Social role relationship lies between the addresser and addressee, it could be either symmetrical (equal status) or asymmetrical (imbalanced status or some form of authority). Social attitude, meanwhile, is the formality or informality of a text and can be judged from the degree of social distance or proximity. Finally, the dimension of Province is, House admits, broadly defined as the "area of operation" of the language activity, which could be derived anywhere from the text producer's occupational and professional activities to the field or topic of the text (ibid., p. 30). In this chapter, we highlight the relevant dimensions of language use from our findings, based on the MQM model.

We evaluated the Medium of the text at its syntactic, lexical, and textual levels. According to House (1977/1981, p. 45), "if a translation text, in order to be adequate, is to fulfil the requirement of a dimensional, and as a result of this, a functional match, then any mismatch along the dimensions is an error." The syntactic level of the evaluation text in Chinese consists of expanded subordinate clauses before the main clauses, which are typical structures in the written mode, and the pervasive use of expanded post-modification which separates the head of the subject noun phrase from the relative clauses. The complex syntactic structures make it difficult for the NMT model to translate the original correctly in the output. For example, in the segment 与 "新型冠状病毒感染的肺炎诊疗方案 (试行)"中推荐的洛匹那韦, 利托那韦, 利巴韦林相比, 山柰酚, 槲皮素, 木犀草素显示出相似的结合能力 [*yu "xin xing guan zhuang bing du gan ran de fei yan zhen liao fang an (shi xing)" zhong tui jian de luo pi na wei, li tuo na wei, li ba wei lin xiang bi, shan nai fen, hu pi su, mu xi cao su xian shi chu xiang si de jie he neng li*], the complex syntactic structure of the list of different names of Western medicines and Chinese herbal ingredients confused the NMT model, resulting in a mistranslation: "compared to lopinavir, ritonavir, and ribavirin, which are recommended in the coronavirus pneumonia treatment protocol for novel coronavirus infection (trial), showed similar binding ability." At the lexical level, although the Chinese original has a few modal adverbials and subjective markers, genre-specific terminologies are pervasive. In House's (1997) model, the register covers three main elements (Field, Tenor, and Mode), of which Field refers to the subject matter and social action of the text and covers the specificity of lexical items. Due to the limited availability of domain-specific data and resources, the NMT model was mostly unable to produce equivalent terms in the translation for terms in the field of TCM, resulting in several terminological mismatches. At the textual level, the source text itself is marked by elaborateness and explicitness in the written mode although the textual level of the evaluation text contains some references to the addresser and the addressee, mostly appearing in quotations of secondary sources, such as 明代张三锡"医学六要"云:"湿令流行,民多寒疫" [*ming dai zhang san xi "yi xue liu yao" yun: "shi ling liu xiang, min duo han yi"*] (Chang San Xi, The Six Key Concepts in Medicine Studies in Ming dynasty, "During the wet seasons, people easily get affected by the cold pandemic").

In the dimension of Participation, the source text is directly addressed, with few personal or possessive pronouns. In the present study, 5 out of 1,405 sample segments used the Chinese personal pronouns 我们 [*wo men*] (we). In fact, the use of first-person personal pronouns is often accepted in academic writing when seeking to produce active and engaging narratives, but beyond occasional use, the source text lacks the explicit involvement of the addresser and addressee. This is reflected in the MT version, whose participation dimension accords with the original.

In the dimension of Social attitude, we discovered that the MT output has very few informal instances, consistent with our analysis of the source text, which is more distant and had a structure with less addressee involvement. Some mismatch errors could still be found in the translation, however, such as 凡入吴蜀地游宦, 体上常须两三处灸之, 勿令疮暂瘥, 瘴疠温疟毒气不能著人也 [*fan ru wu shu di you huan, ti shang chang xu liang san chu jiu zhi, wu ling chuang zan chai, zhang li wen nue du qi bu neng zhuo ren ye*], which was translated as "whenever you go into the luoshenshan cave for ordinary people, you usually have two or three ointment of medicine in the body, so as not to stir the ill, and the muti warm and muti venom cannot be told." This translation was categorised as a Mistranslation in our analysis, but it is interesting to note that the use of "you" to replace 宦 [*huan*] (official) in the translation makes the target text more personal and thus less socially distanced and informal for a scientific paper.

Another essential aspect to be analysed in House's model is the situation's contextual features—the "situational dimensions" (1997, p. 37). This signifies that the analysis of the textual function of a given text should be based on the functional equivalence between the source text and the target text. The function of the text consists of two components—ideational and interpersonal—which are defined as follows:

> a) "to inform the addressees of a collection of facts as precisely and efficiently as possible and to request action";
>
> b) "to establish a positive rapport with the addressees, to convince and reassure them of the appropriateness and advantages of certain moves by the company, to give the addressees a feeling of importance and power, and at the same time to always attempt to be indirect and non-committal as to the moves announced and their potential consequences" (House 2015, p. 48).

The ideational component of the text's textual functions predominates, with condensed information in the written mode, because scientific facts are used in the original to convey facts without the presence of rhetoric of both addressers and addressees. Considering this textual function, omission of any addressee-involving structures would be expected, but the segment 至唐代孙思邈提出 "屠苏酒" 以 "辟邪气, 令人不染温病" [*zhi tang dai sun si miao ti chu "tu su jiu" yi "pi xie qi, ling ren bu ran wen bing"*] for example was translated as "to the end of the tang dynasty, sun yat-sen proposed 'slaughter and wine' to 'rule out the evil, let's not catch the warm disease'" in the MT version. The contraction "let's" suggests a call-to-action for both the addresser and the addressee, which involves making a request to the addressee and is a more interpersonal component of the textual function.

The analysis of the source text and the translation by human assessors revealed mismatches in Field, Tenor, and Mode, with support from the MQM model for more detailed error taxonomies. Regarding Field, the inadequacy of the NMT model in translating TCM terminologies made the MT version less accurate. For Tenor, the author's stance was changed occasionally, meaning that the NMT model was inconsistent in adopting an appropriate written academic genre. For Mode, the original rarely required addressee-involving structures due to its written form, and the translation was mostly in line with this ideational function. If the translation were assessed solely using House's TQA model, we would probably not have identified as many errors as with the MQM model. We can therefore say that, with regard to translation quality assessment, while BLEU cannot determine what the errors are, it can be supplemented by adopting both House's TQA model and Lommel's MQM model.

5. Conclusion

Some of the errors produced by the NMT model could have alarming effects and dire consequences, like mistranslating "feeling cold" as "disgusting cold" or mistranslating the symptoms observed if a person is infected with COVID-19, such as "shortness of breath in the lung" as "first make the lung" and "mild headache" as "micro-ache." This is critical information concerning the symptoms of COVID-19, as an incorrect translation could result in misunderstandings or treatment delays.

Machine translation has drastically increased the volume of translations in recent years, but at critical times, such as during the outbreak of COVID-19, we may find that we have placed too much faith in MT to help in translating a large volume of texts into numerous languages in a short period of time. Even though the BLEU score (22.3) of the machine-translated text for this project might seem acceptable, a more detailed analysis of the errors identified by the two assessors reveals that the accuracy of the MT left something to be desired. The evaluation metrics of BLEU for assessing similarities in the data are clearly inadequate and do not identify the problems themselves. The aims and objectives of MQM—to annotate and categorise errors in the hope of improving the quality of MT—are admirable, but the categorisation of the errors needs to be more refined. Evaluation metrics should include categories at discourse levels, such as pragmatic, semantic, and generic accuracy, which can be explained by House's TQA model.

Given the present study's constrained setting and limited access to only monolingual, target-domain-specific data to supplement the generic parallel data, we concede that the result of this study is not representative of an industrial setting. Indeed, the limitations of this study highlight pertinent problems, such as the costliness of data for research on MT and the non-humanistic and non-culturally-sensitive nature of MT. Algorithms for MT are well suited to statistics and the regularity of language, but the nuances of communication at the discourse, pragmatic, and social levels are better understood and rendered by humans. Therefore, to avoid relying solely on MT, an improved model of human-intervened MT is necessary.

Acknowledgment

This paper was supported by the 2019/20 General Research Fund: When AI Meets TCM: Neural Machine Translating Traditional Chinese Medicine Texts (Project Number: 12600519), sponsored by RGC during the period January 1, 2020 to December 31, 2021.

Wayne Wen-chun Liang is Associate Professor in Translation, Soochow University, Taiwan. Wayne's research interests include literary translation, sociology of translation, translation of regional literature, and machine translation. He has published in international venues, including *Perspectives*, *Babel*, and *mTm*.

Ester S.M. Leung is Associate Professor of Translation Studies (Chinese), University of Melbourne. Ester researches legal and medical interpreting studies using action research approaches. She has published in international journals such as *International Journal for the Semiotics of Law, Multilingua*, and *Interpreting*. Her impact research has received a world-leading (4*) ranking.

Chun-Hin Tse is a PhD candidate researching non-autoregressive neural machine translation at Hong Kong Baptist University. As the senior research assistant, he managed the data collection, pre-processing for the model training, and machine evaluation for this project.

References

Amancio, R. Diego, Maria das Graças Volpe Nunes, Osvaldo N Oliveira, T.A.S. Pardo, L. Antiqueira and Luciano da F. Costa. 2011. "Using metrics from complex networks to evaluate machine translation." *Physica A: Statistical Mechanics and Its Applications* 390, no. 1: 131–142.
Bassnett, Susan. 2003. *Translation Studies.* London: Routledge.

Dunder, Ivan, Sanja Seljan, and Marko Pavlovski. 2020. "Automatic machine translation of poetry and a low-resource language pair." *43rd International Convention on Information, Communication and Electronic Technology (MIPRO)*, 1034–1039.

Gentzler, Edwin. 2017. *Translation and Rewriting in the Age of Post-Translation Studies*. New York: Routledge.

Hassan, Hany, Anthony Aue, Chang Chen, Vishal Chowdhary, Jonathan Clark, Christian Federmann, Xuedong Huang et al. 2018. *Achieving Human Parity on Automatic Chinese to English News Translation*. Accessed June 18, 2021. http://arxiv.org/abs/1803.05567.

House, Juliane. 1977/1981. *A Model for Translation Quality Assessment*. Tübingen: G. Narr.

House, Juliane. 1997. *Translation Quality Assessment: a Model Revisited*. Tübingen: G. Narr.

House, Juliane. 2001. "Translation quality assessment: Linguistic description versus social evaluation." *Meta* 46, no. 2: 243–257.

House, Juliane. 2009. *Translation*. Oxford: Oxford University Press.

House, Juliane. 2015. *Translation Quality Assessment: Past and Present*. London: Routledge.

Jin, Di, Zhijing Jin, Joey Tianyi Zhou, and Peter Szolovits. 2020. A Simple Baseline to Semi-Supervised Domain Adaptation for Machine Translation. Manuscript accessed on June 18, 2021. https://doi.org/10.48550/arXiv.2001.08140.

Lample, Guillaume, and Alexis Conneau. 2019. *Cross-lingual Language Model Pretraining*. Accessed June 18, 2021. https://doi.org/10.48550/arXiv.1901.07291.

Lommel, Arle, Aljoscha Burchardt, Maja Popović, Kim Harris, Eleftherios Avramidis, and Hans Uszkoreit. 2014. "Using a new analytic measure for the annotation and analysis of MT errors on real data." *Proceedings of the 17th Annual Conference of the European Association for Machine Translation (EAMT 2014)*. Accessed August 18, 2021. https://www.dfki.de/fileadmin/user_upload/import/7426_Lommel_el_al_2014_MQM.pdf.

Mutua, Makau. 2001. "Savages, victims, and saviors: The metaphor of human rights." *Harvard International Law Journal* 42, no. 1: 201–245.

Papineni, Kishore, Salim Roukos, Todd Ward, and Wei-Jing Zhu. 2002. "BLEU: a method for automatic evaluation of machine translation." *Proceedings of the 40th Annual Meeting on Association for Computational Linguistics (ACL '02)*. Accessed August 16, 2021. https://doi.org/10.3115/1073083.1073135.

Popović, Maja. 2018. "Error Classification and Analysis for Machine Translation Quality Assessment." In *Translation Quality Assessment: from Principles to Practice*, edited by Joss Moorkens, Sheila Castilho, Federico Gaspari, and Stephen Doherty. Dordrecht: Springer International Publishing AG, 129–158.

Reiss, Katharina. 1989. "Text types, translation types and translation assessment." In *Readings in Translation Theory*, edited by Andrew Chesterman, 105–115. Helsinki: Oy Finn Lectura Ab.

Saldanha, Gabriela, and Sharon O'Brien. 2014. *Research Methodologies in Translation Studies*. Manchester: Routledge.

Seljan, Sanja, and Ivan Dunder. 2015a. "Automatic quality evaluation of machine-translated output in sociological-philosophical-spiritual domain." *10th Iberian Conference on Information Systems and Technologies (CISTI)*, 1–4.

Seljan, Sanja, and Ivan Dunder. 2015b. "Machine translation and automatic evaluation of English/Russian-Croatian." *International Conference «Corpus Linguistics – 2015» (CORPORA 2015)*, 72–79.

Seljan, Sanja, Marko Tucaković, and Ivan Dunder. 2015. "Human evaluation of online machine translation services for English/Russian-Croatian." *3rd World Conference on Information Systems and Technologies (WorldCIST'15)*. Dordrecht: Springer International Publishing AG.

Sennrich, Rico, Barry Haddow, and Alexandra Birch. 2016. "Improving neural machine translation models with monolingual data." *Proceedings of the 54th Annual Meeting of the Association for Computational Linguistics (Volume 1: Long Papers).* Berlin, Germany, 86–96.

Shiffman, Daniel. 2012. *The Nature of Code: Simulating Natural Systems with Processing.* Accessed June 19, 2021. http://natureofcode.com/.

Vaswani, Ashwin, Samy Bengio, Eugene Brevdo, Francois Chollet, Aidan N. Gomez, Stephan Gouws, Llion Jones, Łukasz Kaiser, Nal Kalchbrenner, Niki Parmar, Ryan Sepassi, Noam Shazeer, and Jakob Uszkoreit. 2018. *Tensor2tensor for Neural Machine Translation.* Accessed August 18, 2021. https://arxiv.org/abs/1803.07416.

Appendix 1. Annotators' (Human Intervened) Evaluations based on 1,405 Sample Segments

Error	Frequency	Examples
Accuracy		
Terminology	265	黃連解毒湯 [huang lian jie du tang] (yellow powder decoction) 雙黃蓮口服液 [shuang huang lian kou fu ye] (Dual-luoro-adhesive oral fluid) 新冠肺炎 [xin guan fei yan] (new crown pneumonia)
Omission	19	1.4 麻黃—蒼術治療新冠肺炎的潛在靶點預測 [1.4 ma huang—cang zhu zhi liao xin guan fei yan de qian zai ba dian yu ce] (1.4 prediction of potential targets for the treatment of new coronavirus) 中国工程院钟南山院士接受新华社专访时亦指出，COVID-19确诊患者当中发热仍是最主要的和最典型的症状[16] [zhong guo gong cheng yuan zhong nan shan yuan shi jie shou xin hua she zhuan fang shi yi zhi chu, COVID-19 que zhen huan zhe dang zhong fa re reng shi zui zhu yao de he zui dian xing de zheng zhuang [16]] (the chinese university of hong kong, when the chinese university of hong kong, received special attention from xinhua university, also noted that fever remained the most predominant and typical symptom among covid-19 confirmed patients [16].)

Error	Frequency	Examples
Mistranslation	408	不是通过具体的"望, 闻, 问, 切" 手段 辨证, 而是建立在对所有已患病者证的综合分析基础之上得到的方案 [bu shi tong guo ju ti de "wang, wen, wen, qie" shou duan bian zheng, er shi jian li zai dui suo you yi huan bing zhe zheng de zong he fen xi ji chu zhi shang de dao de fang an] (rather than discerning through the specific "hope, smell, ask, cut" means, the scheme that builds upon the comprehensive analysis of all the sick person's certificates is)
		另外 , 从临床表现来看, 新冠肺炎患者重型, 危重型患者病程中可为中, 低热, 甚至无明显发热 [ling wai, cong lin chuang biao xian lai kan, xin guan fei yan huan zhe zhong xing, wei zhong xing huan zhe bing cheng zhong ke wei zhong, di re, shen zhi wu ming xian fa re] (in addition, in terms of clinical manifestations, severe, low-grade fever in patients with new coronavirus-induced pneumonia and even no significant fever)
		中药配方颗粒, 沸水冲服, 每日2次[广东一方制药有限公司生产, 许可证号(粤) 20160214, 产品批号9115313] [zhong yao pei fang ke li, fei shui chong fu, mei ri 2 ci [guang dong yi fang zhi yao you xian gong si sheng chan, xu ke zheng hao (yue) 20160214, chan pin pi hao 9115313]] (chinese medicine formulation pellets, boiling water rinse, twice daily [guangdong one pharmaceutical co., ltd., production no. (guangdong) 20160214, product batch no. 9115313])
		2.1.2 药物归经与性味分析 [yao wu gui jing yu xing wei fen xi] (2.1.2 drug repurposing: drug repurposing with sexual taste analysis)
Untranslated	0	
Addition	0	
Fluency		
Spelling	5	2.7 阿比朵爾[a bi duo er(arbidol)](2.7 abbidol (arbidol))
		接下来 , 武汉病毒研究所石正丽团队又用实验进一步证实 ace 2 确实对于新型冠状病毒感染细胞是必需的 [jie xia lai, wu han bing du yan jiu suo shi zheng li tuan dui you yong shi yan jin yi bu zheng shi ace2 que shi dui yu xin xing guan zhuang bing du gan ran xi bao shi bi xu de] (next, the wuhan institute of virology, nishizhuang team further confirmed that ace2 is indeed essential for the generation of novel coronavirus infected cells using experiments)

Error	Frequency	Examples
Typography	1	中医师在美国行医的原则应该是安全第一, 疗效是第二位的[zhong yi shi zai mei guo xing yi de yuan ze ying gai shi an quan di yi, liao xiao shi di er wei de] (the principle of physician practice in the <u>ed</u> should be safe first, with efficacy second)
Grammar	58	Part of speech: 2. 苦参抗冠状病毒的可能作用机制 [2. ku shen kang guan zhuang bing du de ke neng zuo yong ji zhi] (2. the possible mechanism of action of bitter ginseng against coronavirus) Tense/aspect/mood: 2017年, 世界卫生组织报道全球每年有近3000万的患者罹患此病, 病死率高达 50% ~ 70% [12-13] [2017 nian, shi jie wei sheng zu zhi bao dao quan qiu mei nian you jin 3000 wan de huan zhe li huan ci bing, bing si lü gao da 50%~70%[12-13]] (in 2017, the world health organization reported that nearly 30 million patients worldwide suffer from the disease every year, with morbidity rates as high as 50 % to 70 % [12-13].) 死亡比率下降除与医疗资源显著改善相关外, 适当的抗病毒治疗和中医药物使用, 也可能发挥了一定作用 [si wang bi lü xia jiang chu yu yi liao zi yuan xian zhu gai shan xiang guan wai, shi dang de kang bing du zhi liao he zhong yi yao wu shi yong, ye ke neng fa hui le yi ding zuo yong] (the decrease in the death ratio, in addition to its correlation with significant improvement in medical resources, appropriate antiviral therapy and the use of traditional chinese medicine may also play a role) 据世界卫生组织(WHO)不完全统计, 人类历史上曾爆发了天花、黑死病(学名"鼠疫")、艾滋病、登革热与西尼罗热、非典(严重急性呼吸综合征, SARS)、霍乱、埃博拉、血吸虫病、禽流感和脊髓灰质炎(又称"小儿麻痹症")等10大传染病疫情扩散事件 [ju shi jie wei sheng zu zhi (WHO) bu wan quan tong ji, ren lei li shi shang ceng bao fa le tian hua, hei si bing (xue ming "shu yi"), ai zi bing, deng ge re yu xi ni luo re, fei dian (yan zhong ji xing hu xi zong he zheng, SARS), huo luan, ai bo la, xue xi chong bing, qin liu gan he ji sui hui zhi yan (you cheng "xiao er ma bi zheng") deng 10 da chuan ran bing yi qing kuo san shi jian] (according to the world health organization (who), human history has been a major outbreak of smallpox, black death (known as "plague"), hiv, dengue and west nile fever, aids (severe acute respiratory syndrome, sars), cholera, ebola, schistosomiasis, avian influenza, and poliomyelitis (also known as "polio").)

Error	Frequency	Examples
		Word order:
		自2月12日开始国家卫健委网站单独公布武汉新型冠状病毒肺炎病例数据, 且数据采集中所需数据资料完整 [zi 2 yue 12 ri kai shi guo jia wei jian wei wang zhan dan du gong bu wu han xin xing guan zhuang bing du fei yan bing li shu ju, qie shu ju cai ji zhong suo xu shu ju zi liao wan zheng] (since february 12, the national guard website released data on cases of novel coronavirus pneumonia in wuhan separately, and the data availability required in data collection is complete)
		2.3.1 不同使用频次的中药对COVID-19疾病网络稳健性的扰动分析[2.3.1 bu tong shi yong pin ci de zhong yao dui COVID-19 ji bing wang luo wen jian xing de rao dong fen xi] (2.3.1 perturbation analysis of the COVID-19 disease network robustness of different use of medium)
		Incorrect function words:
		与先前爆发的sars 冠状病毒 (sars-cov) 及中东呼吸综合征冠状病毒 (mers-cov)相比 , 新型冠状病毒除了具有相似的基因组, 体内复制动力学和生物学性质外 , 还表现出一些独特性 [3, 4] [yu xian qian bao fa de sars guan zhuang bing du sars-cov) ji zhong dong hu xi zong he zheng guan zhuang bing du (mers-cov) xiang bi, xin xing guan zhuang bing du chu le ju you xiang si de ji yin zu, ti nei fu zhi dong li xue he sheng wu xue xing zhi wai, hai biao xian chu yi xie du te xing [3, 4]] (in contrast to previous outbreaks of sars coronavirus (sars-cov) and middle east respiratory syndrome coronavirus (mers-cov), the novel coronavirus exhibits some uniqueness in addition to its similar genome, in vivo replication kinetics, and biological properties [3, 4].)
		2. 湖北与武汉新增确诊及新增死亡病例的变化曲线 [2. hu bei yu wu han xin zeng que zhen ji xin zeng si wang bing li de bian hua qu xian] (2. the curve of the change in new confirmed and new deaths in hubei <u>with</u> wuhan)
Unintelligible	47	2.2 连花清瘟的抗炎抑菌作用和炎症风暴 [2.2 lian hua qing wen de kang yan yi jun zuo yong he yan zheng feng bao] (2.2 anti-inflammatory and inflammatory storms of streptococcus spp . , streptococcus spp . , streptococcus spp . , streptococcus spp . , streptococcus spp . ,)
		2.3 莲花清瘟治疗2019-ncov潜在作用靶点[2.3 lian hua qing wen zhi liao 2019-ncov qian zai zuo yong ba dian] (2.3purpurpurpurpurpurpurpurpurpurpurpurpur-purpurpurpurpurpurpurpurpurpurpurpurpur-purpurpurpurpurpurpurpurpur)

CHAPTER 4

From "Selfless Hospitality" to "Get Out": Disrupting the 2020 Games

Claire Maree

Abstract

In this chapter the author explores how disruptions caused by the ongoing COVID-19 pandemic have created tensions and clashes with the 2020 Tokyo Olympic Games' vision of "Unity in Diversity" and "United by Emotion," as seen in increasing xenophobia and protest against the Games. It is argued that the polite undertones of "selfless hospitality" (*omotenashi*) resonate with the impolite demands to "get out" in a way which demonstrates the fragile nature of *omotenashi* as an act of un/welcoming the foreign.

Keywords: im/politeness, hospitality, *omotenashi*, Tokyo 2020 Olympic and Paralympic Games, anti-Olympic protests, framing

1. Introduction

The 2020 Olympic and Paralympic Games, (hereafter 2020 Games) were postponed to the Northern Hemisphere summer of 2021 as a result of the ongoing COVID-19 pandemic.[1] The conceptual welcoming of visitors to Japan which was mobilised through the notion of おもてなし [*omotenashi*] (hospitality) in the 2013 bid for the 2020 Games took on a decidedly "unwelcoming" turn as Tokyo and the surrounding areas entered a fourth period of state of emergency prior to the Opening Ceremony (July 23, 2021). An anti-Olympic movement had been active since the bidding stage (Holthus et al., 2020), but dissatisfaction grew even more acute as the domestic medical system came under great stress, a large percentage of the population were yet to be vaccinated, and borders remained closed to many non-Japanese residents. Reports of anti-Olympic protests appeared in the mainstream press globally as IOC members began to assemble for the Opening Ceremony and protestors gathered at key sites. The hashtag #バッハ帰れ [*#Bachkaere*] (#getoutBach) gained traction on social media.

Politeness and impoliteness are situated evaluations (Haugh, 2013, pp. 8–9; Davies et al., 2013) which are enacted within localised ideologies (Dunn, 2011; Eelen, 2001; Mills, 2003; Pizziconi, 2006). The *omotenashi* discourse emerging from the 2013 bid mobilises politeness in the preparation and staging of a mega-event, the hashtag activism using imperatives such as *#Bachkaere* mobilises impoliteness to contradict the polite posturing of the official discourse. Although very different genres, both campaigns mobilise im/politeness as a pivotal component and exploit social norms of what is, and how to be, polite (Watts, 1992; Jary, 1998, Ohashi, 2008).

In this chapter, I demonstrate how the rhetoric of "selfless hospitality"—one of the translations provided for the term *omotenashi* used in the bidding process, which framed the Olympic discourse in the planning stages—is disrupted by the COVID-19 pandemic, and furthermore how disruptions caused by the COVID-19 pandemic discombobulate local and global communities exhorted by the 2020 Games official motto to be "united by emotion." In response to the staging of the 2020 Games during a time of crisis, anti-Olympic activists reframe the polite undertones of *omotenashi* through strategic use of impolite terms such as 帰れ [*kaere*] (go home) circulated on social media and cited in street protests.

The discourse of *omotenashi* emerges from official promotional materials. The discourse of *kaere* emerges from anti-Olympic protest movements. Both, however, can be viewed as slogans which clash in the lead up to the postponed Games. This clash reveals that, in the face of a global pandemic in which borders are closed except to a privileged few, "selfless hospitality" is an impossibility.

2. The Recovery Games

The 2020 Tokyo Olympic and Paralympic Games are the second summer Olympics to be held in Japan.[2] The first Tokyo summer Games in 1964 were held a little over a decade after Japan's defeat in the Second World War and subsequent occupation by the USA. In 1964, the nation sought to re-establish and rebrand itself as a liberal democracy and player in the contemporary global economy. It did so through cultural diplomacy which incorporated global Olympic values, and a discourse of "harmony" (Collins, 2011). Five decades later, the bid for the 2020 Games was couched in soft-diplomacy rhetoric of "Cool Japan" as Japan emerged, not from colonising warfare, but the devastation of the Great East Japan Earthquake (2011). The 9.0-magnitude earthquake caused a tsunami which resulted in the crippling of the Fukushima nuclear power plant. The Fukushima Daiichi Nuclear Accident measured Level 7 on the International Nuclear Event Scale and was a cause of ongoing concern that necessitated mitigation in the context of the bid for the 2020 Games.

Positioned as the 復興五輪 [*fukkō gorin*] or "Recovery Olympics," the Reconstruction Agency of Japan notes on its English-language website that the 2020 Games represents an opportunity to "boost ... the reconstruction of the regions affected" (n.d.). The website endorses the transformative power of the Olympics, proclaiming that "the Tokyo 1964 Games completely changed Japan" and that the 2020 Games will be "the most innovative in history." The cancellation of the 1940 Olympics due to the encroaching war is obfuscated by referring to "the prevailing international situation at the time" which "resulted in the cancellation." The website goes on to claim that the "objective behind the original bid to host the 1940 Games" was "to showcase to a global audience the great progress Japan had made since opening up to the world in 1868, and Tokyo's recovery and reconstruction from the devastation of the Great Kanto Earthquake in 1923." The re-employment of "peacefulness" in the context of the 1964 Olympics hinges on the guise of the Olympics' claim to being apolitical (Droubie, 2011). Although not cancelled, the global pandemic would eventually force the postponement until 2021 of what would still be referred to as the "2020" Games.

The 2020 Games are grounded in "diversity" and "unity" which emanate from the overarching Olympic value of "unity in diversity" espoused in IOC President Bach's 2013 manifesto. The concepts of "unity," diversity," and "hospitality" are not unique to the 2020 Games, and were mobilised, for example, as conceptual frameworks in the 2012 London Olympics and Paralympics (Hubbard and Wilkinson, 2015). Practices of resemiotisation (Iedema, 2001, 2003; Oostendorp, 2018) transpose concepts of diversity and inclusion into culturally and socio-politically legible local initiatives and campaigns. Such local initiatives and campaigns demonstrate alignment with Olympic values and also position the host city—and by connection the nation and its people—within contemporary global geopolitics. One example is the東京都オリンピック憲章にうたわれる人権尊重の理念の現実を目指す条例 [*Tōkyōto orinpikku kenshō ni utawareru jinken sonchō no rinen no genjitsu o mezasu jōrei*] (Tokyo Municipal Ordinance with the aim of realising the values of respect for human rights as extolled in the Olympic Charter) which was adopted by the Tokyo Municipal Government in 2018. The ordinance aligns with the IOC's non-discrimination clause and is aimed at promoting awareness for the rights of sexual minorities and denouncing hate speech against ethnic and sexual minorities. The ordinance notions towards the type of "diversity" envisioned as critical to the 2020 Games. As there are few real ramifications for individuals and corporations who do not uphold this spirit of awareness raising, it also betrays the limitations of such diversity measures.

The aspirational goals contained in initiatives are articulated through slogans and mottos. These short, catchy phrases which are formulated to encapsulate abstract concepts appear on official Olympic announcements, media communications, and marketing paraphernalia. Multiple modes such as colour, sound, and/or camera angle are collaboratively manipulated in the writing, design, and editing of these emblems, mottos, and slogans, which frame (Goffman, 1974; Butler, 2009) the planning and staging of the mega-event. Used in incremental steps, logos and emblems simultaneously orient to both the mega-event and the promise of its ongoing legacy. Positive legacy building (Girginov and Hills, 2008) is a key testament of the planning and delivery of contemporary Olympic Games.

In this chapter I focus on the term *omotenashi* (lit. hospitality) which, like "diversity" and "unity" is co-opted into 2020 Games discourse and functions much like a slogan. I trace the term to a speech delivered as part of the 2013 Bid and unpack the complex translatory processes by which it has been rendered as a "uniquely Japanese" form of hospitality steeped in notions of politeness. Commodified, marketed, and sold as part of the proposed 2020 Games experience, this "unique" form of Japanese hospitality acts as a "frame." Social frameworks, Goffman notes, "provide background understanding for events that incorporate the will, aim, and controlling effort of an intelligence" (Goffman, 1974, p. 22). The frame of *omotenashi* underlines the controlling effort of the host city to market the Games as welcoming in a uniquely Japanese manner. The frame of *omotenashi* becomes unhinged in the face of disruption caused by a global pandemic; use of the decidedly un/welcoming hashtag *#Bachkaere* (getoutBach) in social media activism and the citation of the hashtag in placards used at protests underlines the problematics of "selflessly" "welcoming" visitors during a public-health crisis at a time when borders remained closed to many. Before we turn to an analysis of the disruption, let us first look towards mobilisation of this initial *omotenashi* framing in the 2013 Bid process.

3. The Global and the Foreign in the Performance of *Omotenashi*

The framing of the 2020 Games in the rhetoric of *omotenashi* hospitality can be traced back to the speech delivered in French by Takigawa Christel (Masami Christel Takigawa Lardux 1977–) as part of the final bid presented at the IOC General Business meeting in Buenos Aires in 2013. A former news anchor and freelance announcer noted for her bilingual skills, Takigawa was appointed as a "Cool Tokyo" Ambassador to take "a lead role in promoting the dynamic and vibrant culture in the heart of one of the world's most exciting cities" (The Tokyo Organising Committee of the Olympic and Paralympic Games website) in June 2013. The speech promising unique Japanese hospitality delivered in French anchors the bid within localised discourses of the global. As a bilingual personality, Takigawa functions as conduit for notions of hospitality which can be translated into languages other than

Japanese. As a bicultural personality, Takigawa functions as a symbolic trace of the foreign welcomed into Japan who can be made to feel un/welcome.

Delivered in French and prefaced by a short address from Inose Naoki (then Governor of Tokyo; Chair of Tokyo 2020), Takigawa's speech reinforces the merits of staging the mega-event in Tokyo. The speech promises that Japan will "offer you a unique welcome," known as *omotenashi* (Transcript 1, lines 1–2). Warmly smiling and with pinched hand to the side of her shoulder, Takigawa slowly articulates each syllable of the phrase *o-mo-te-na-shi* as she gently moves her hand across the space in front of her torso. Pausing slightly on each syllable, Takigawa releases her fingers into an open sidewards palm on the final *shi* (Example 1, line 2) after which she brings her palms together. Eyes closed Takigawa bows on the final *omotenashi* (Example 1, line 2). *Omotenashi*, Takigawa explains, "dates back to our ancestors" (Transcript 1, line 4) yet can be found in "Japan's ultra-modern culture" (Transcript 1, line 5). It is key to "why Japanese people take care of each other, and our guests" (Transcript 1, line 6) so well. Takigawa proffers the example of lost money being returned to police as an example of this uniquely Japanese spirit. After introducing the concept of *omotenashi*, the speech goes on to stress the safety of the city, and the culinary and shopping opportunities which can be enjoyed alongside the consumption of the Games.

> Transcript 1. Takigawa's speech in French with English (September 11, 2013 NHK)
>
> 1. Nous vous offrirons un accueil vraiment unique.
>
> (We will offer you a unique welcome.)
>
> 2. En japonais, il est possible de le décrire avec un seul mot : o-mo-te-na-shi.
>
> (In Japanese, I can describe it in one unique word: omotenashi.)
>
> 3. L'omotenashi, c'est un sens profond de l'hospitalité, généreux et désintéressé...
>
> (It means a spirit of selfless hospitality...)
>
> 4. Qui remonte à l'époque de nos ancêtres...
>
> (One that dates back to our ancestors...)
>
> 5. Et qui est depuis resté ancré dans la culture ultra-moderne du Japon.
>
> (Yet is ingrained in Japan's ultra-modern culture.)
>
> 6. Cet « Omotenashi » explique pourquoi les Japonais prennent autant soin les uns des autres, de la même façon qu'ils prennent soin de leurs invités.
>
> ("Omotenashi" explains why Japanese people take care of each other... and our guests... so well.)

As work on politeness emphasises, im/politeness is evaluated in specific localised contexts (Eelen, 2001; Dunn, 2006, 2013; Pizzicconi, 2006). In the case of this speech, we can identify two local contexts which co-occur. One is the immediate context of a delivery to a global audience in French. This co-occurs with a second context of a display oriented to Japanese audiences for whom the delivery is interpreted simultaneously and also translated into texts to be reported in Japanese. Both the performative act of speaking in French, and the translation into Japanese are relevant to our discussion. Furthermore, as politeness is a "multimodal semiotic register" (Dunn, 2018, p. 17) the use of language and the body are important here: Takigawa's gestures are a key component of the *omotenashi* framing.

First, let us consider the Japanese phrase *omotenashi*, which is a combination of the beautification and/or honorific particle *o*, and the noun *motenashi*. Shogakukan's Japanese Dictionary, the largest dictionary of its kind for Japanese, lists five meanings for *motenashi*. The second listed meaning is: 人に対する態度。人に対するふるまい方。人に対する遇し方。待遇。[*Hito ni taisuru taido. Hito ni taisuru furumai-kata. Hito ni taisuru gūshi-kata. Taigū*] (Attitudes to people. Conduct/way of behaving towards people. Way of treating people. Treatment), and the fifth is 饗応。ごちそう。[*kyōō, gochisō*] (entertaining [with food and drink]. Entertainment; a dinner and/or a feast). Turning to Shogakukan's *Progressive Japanese-French Dictionary*, the possible translations for the verb *motenasu* provided are: *accueillir* (welcome), *recevoir* (to receive [welcome]), *donner l'hospitalité* (give hospitality). The description Takigawa offers in the speech in French is: "*un sens profond de l'hospitalité, généreux et désintéressé.*" Although the NHK renders this as "a spirit of selfless hospitality" (Transcript 1, line 3) we could translate as "a spirit of hospitality, generous and selfless."

The Japanese national broadcaster NHK published both Japanese translations for the speeches along with the video which includes an English translation for Takigawa's speech (Transcription 1). As noted above, the English translation (Transcript 1, line 3) for the definition of *omotenashi* in French is "a spirit of selfless hospitality." The entry in the largest Japanese to English dictionary, *New Kenkyusha Japanese-English Dictionary*, explains that "treatment" and/or "reception" is in reference to "guests," and henceforth the term can be used to mean "service." "Entertainment" and "sumptuous meals," as well as "welcome," "entertainment," and "hospitality" are listed as possible equivalents for the notion of "treatment." Even with the addition of the honorific and/or beautification particle *o*, it would be difficult to make a case for the inclusion of "selflessness" in a direct translation of *omotenashi* into English.

The Japanese translation provided by NHK underlines the semantic shift which is undergone by offering the explanatory phrase: 見返りを求めないホスピタリティの精神 [*mikaeri o motomenai hosupitaritī no seishin*]. Here, "(a) spirit of hospitality" (*hosupitaritī no seishin*) is modified by the phrase "*mikaeri o motomenai*" which we could translate as "(that) for/in which return favours are not sought." *Omotenashi* could then be rendered as "a spirit of hospitality in which return favours are not sought."

Takigawa's speech as part of the 2013 bid is an example of what Dunn refers to as aesthetic labour (Dunn, 2018). As deportment and use of appropriate honorific language indexes not only appropriate business conduct, but also respectability (Dunn, 2018; Pizziconi, 2007), we could thus interpret the final bow Takigawa performs as a refined embodiment of business conduct; an appropriate gesture with which to animate an invitation to people around the world to visit Japan once Tokyo secures its place as the host city. Although bows and bowing constitute both business conduct and aesthetic labour, the bringing of hands together in front of the chest with fingers pointing upwards is not typically part of formal bowing in either business or service encounters in Japan. Rather, it is more commonly used in apologies, or performed in front of a shrine or temple altar as part of respectful religiosity. The final bow here indexes submission which is visually performed by the bringing together of hands which satisfies the orientalising gaze of a global audience. The notion of "selflessness," therefore, is laminated onto "hospitality" through translatory processes and multimodal politeness.

Takigawa's delivery of *omotenashi* accompanied by hand movement and final bow was a celebrated moment repeated across multiple media channels. Takigawa is filmed exiting the customs hall of the international airport on return from Buenos Aires and presented with flowers. The assembled media calls for her to pose. In a live interview recorded by ANN News (September 2013) as she departs the airport, Takigawa stresses how important it was for her to include the concept of *omotenashi* in the speech. Upon being congratulated for the performance, Takigawa is careful to note that it was not of her own design, before obligingly recreating it for the cameras: *o-mo-te-na-shi.*

The self-citation which Takigawa enacts as she exits the airport in 2013 begins a citational chain of mediatisation and commodification. TV news, newspapers, reporters, and comedians alike cite what becomes an iconic media moment. *Omotenashi* is voted one of the four U-can Neologism and Buzzword Award buzz-words of the year in 2013 (for discussion of the significance of this award see Miller, 2017). The photo accompanying the blurb used on the U-can Award website depicts Takigawa leaning out to the side with her hand raised to the side—as if just about to release the final sounds of the now iconic delivery of *o-mo-te-na-shi.*

The gesture is a moment of staged brilliance which has been choreographed to achieve the utmost impact and with an eye to replication, or citation. The cultural concept of *omotenashi* moves further from a dictionary meaning of "welcoming clients and/or guests through provision of entertainment and food" to index a "uniquely Japanese"—and by extrapolation "submissive" and therefore "selfless"— manner of hospitality to be offered to foreign "guests" from abroad. Operating as a frame, *omotenashi* becomes a nostalgic incantation for something "uniquely Japanese" which can be used as a brand to be both celebrated and marketed in the context of the 2020 Games.

4. Commodification of *omotenashi*

As the 2020 Games planning and preparation moved to the next stage, the term *omotenashi* was further commodified. Through processes of commodification, words are made separate from the people who use them (Miller, 2017, p. 45) and *omotenashi* moves from the realm of vernacular speech to function as an overarching principle for welcoming visitors to Japan. For example, the Tokyo Municipal Government commenced the Omotenashi Volunteerism programme. The website invites citizens to "learn about the volunteerism which offers hospitality to many visitors from other countries to Tokyo as the opportunity of the Games" (n.d). An introductory, short English course called the "Omotenashi Course" was offered between 2015 and 2019. The Ministry for Economy, Trade and Industry (METI) introduced in 2017 (revised 2019) an Omotenashi Skills Program: 日本古来のおもてなしの概念を基に [*Nihonkorai no omotenashi no gainen o moto ni*] (based on the time-honoured Japanese concept of hospitality). Note that in both instances, the term "hospitality" is used as a translation for *omotenashi*.

METI's *Omotenashi* ratings include 4 levels—from no stars to three stars. Service providers can apply for one of the ratings. The sliding payment scale includes a one-time registration fee, and annual payments. The starless rating is based on self-designation by the service provider. The three-star rating, however, is based on a detailed index of points for "management" and "inbound" services. The indices for operations and management include such things as regulations around smoking and encouraging "green" and "barrier-free" practices. The inbound checklist includes indices for providing multilingual signage and instructions, alongside facilitation of cultural understanding of the target country. The checklists for achieving accreditation encompass more than traditional etiquette and manners as might be imagined under the rubric of *omotenashi*. This is a hospitality industry grappling with a diversification of clientele within the context of a mega-event governed by an IOC charter which promotes non-discrimination, and a JOC which mobilises "unity in diversity."

5. The Olympics Stall and Opposition Gains Visibility

Resistance to and campaigns against the Olympics are well documented. The anti-Olympic movement has carried out a dedicated global and local campaign for many years (Boykoff, 2014, 2017; Boykoff and Yasuoka, 2014), which is grounded in evidence of the "adverse effects" of mega-sports events (McGillivray, Lauermann, and Turner, 2021, p. 71). New media activism which allows for local issues to be placed in global flows and attain wider attention (Tombleson and Wolf, 2017; Wang and Zhou, 2021) has seen social media activism increasingly mobilised for the cause (McGillivray, Lauermann, and Turner, 2021). As Giulianotti et al. (2015) illustrate in their analysis of critique of the 2012 London Games, a variety of actors motivated by different concerns have expressed dissatisfaction with, and critique of, the Olympics.

Part of a transnational coalition of global activism against the Olympics Games, both the 反五輪の会 [*Hangorin No Kai*] (No Olympics 2020) and オリンピック災害おことわり連絡会 [*Orinpikku-saigai-okotowari-renrakukai*] (No 2020 Olympics Disaster OkotowaLink) mobilised support for the cause through events, public actions and social media platforms. A pamphlet produced by No 2020 Olympics Disaster OkotowaLink outlines twenty reasons to demand that the 2020 Games be cancelled. These include issues which are common to anti-Olympic discourse such as impact on infrastructure, homelessness, the destruction of forests, and bribery. The positioning of the 2020 Games as the "recovery Games" when money which could have been used for recovery and support of those displaced by the 3.11 tragedies was funnelled into construction and other costs is also listed. The 2021 pamphlet includes one additional reason—that of the COVID-19 pandemic. It ends with an impassioned plea for the Games to be cancelled: "To truly put lives first, there is no option but to cancel the Olympics" (2021, n.p.). Nonetheless, the 2020 Games opened in July 2021 as numbers of COVID cases and deaths from the virus soared throughout Japan (*Asahi Shimbun*, 2021) and coincided with Tokyo and surrounding areas entering another period of emergency.

Although the border remained closed to those non-Japanese nationals seeking to re-enter their place of residence and/or study in Japan, competing athletes and teams were granted entry to Japan alongside IOC officials and the press. The frame of "selfless hospitality" which was invoked in the bid, encouraged through volunteerism, and institutionalised through technologies of *omotenashi* rankings became increasingly untenable as public sentiment became decidedly more "unwelcoming." In July 2021, *Asahi* reported that 55% of those surveyed agreed that the Olympics should be cancelled and 68% that the 2020 Games could not be staged in a safe manner as the then Prime Minister Suga maintained. When it became clear that the 2020 Games would go ahead without domestic supporters in the stands, and that the IOC top members would enjoy the luxuries of top-class hotel suites and side trips to Hiroshima, the anti-Olympic movement coordinated online campaigns and demonstrations outside the hotels where key IOC officials resided. Dissatisfaction with the Olympics, and in particular with members of the IOC who visited Japan, took on a new, inhospitable, turn.

Just as guests can be welcomed, so too can they be refused. Within the Japanese hierarchy of politeness, which is enforced through practises of formulaic language, encouragement to depart is more often than not expressed in oblique ways. In the context of growing dissatisfaction with the 2020 Games proceeding during a lockdown, and in particular with the IOC, which is seen to be favouring the mega-event over the public health concerns of the people in the host city, obliqueness is thrown to the wind. Hashtags such as #東京五輪の中止を求めます [*Tokyo gorin no chūshi o motomemasu*] (request the Tokyo Olympics be cancelled) and #バッハ帰れ [*#Bachkaere*] (#getoutBach) gained traction on social media.

Hashtag activism, which Tombleson and Wolf (2017, p. 15) define "as the act of fighting for or supporting a cause with the use of hashtags as primary channel to raise awareness of an issue and encourage debate via social media," makes use of the interconnectivity of metatags (Zappavigna, 2015) to build connected counterpublics (Jackson and Foucault Welles, 2015; Tombleson and Wolf, 2017; Yang, 2016; Xiong, Cho, and Boatwright, 2019). Anti-Olympic activists manipulate norms of politeness and civility in their tags. For example, #五輪の中止を求めます [*gorin no chūshi o motomemasu*] (request the Tokyo Olympics be cancelled) makes use of *motomemasu*, the distal form of the verb *motomeru* (request), and appeals to an unnamed body or institution for the cancellation of the Games. Note, too, that the verb *motomeru* coincidentally appears in the gloss offered by NHK for the translation of Takigawa's 2013 Bid speech cited in the above. However, rather than appealing to ホスピタリティの精神 [*hosupitaritī no seishin*] (a spirit of hospitality), "(that) for/in which return favours are not sought," here it works as a polite demand for cancellation. In contrast, #バッハ帰れ [*Bach kaere*] (go home (or get out) Bach) uses the bold imperative *kaere* (go home) and demands an official of a global mega-event "get out." The impolite demand to *kaere* "get out" is the flip side of *omotenashi* "hospitality," and demonstrates the fragility of un/welcoming the foreign in the context of disruptions to the 2020 Games.

Different norms of politeness co-occur (Haugh, 2013) and incivility and impoliteness are the hallmarks of discourse on social media channels, including those in Japanese (Nishimura, 2019). Although this is often theorised to be a result of the anonymity and detachment common to this media, in a study of reactions to a renowned climate change activist, Andersson (2021) posits that impoliteness and incivility is key to constructing or creating homophilous online communities. In the Japanese socio-political context, as the public loses trust in traditional media in the aftermath of 3.11 (Manabe, 2016; Petrovic, 2020), the culture of anonymity on social media platforms enables dissident social movements to engage in activism and critique. The hashtag *#bachkaere* aligns with 原発やめろ [*genpatsu yamero*] (quit nuclear power) and 安倍やめろ [*Abe yamero*] (quit/resign [Prime Minister] Abe) which emerge from the post-3.11 period.

Both *kaere* (imperative: go home) and *yamero* (imperative: stop) make use of the Japanese imperative form. *Genpatsu yamero* (quit nuclear power) and *Abe yamero* (quit/resign Abe) originate from music and calls made at post-3.11 demonstrations:

the largest protests seen since the anti-ANPO demonstrations of 1960[3] (Manabe, 2016). The Hydrangea Revolution peaked in 2012 (Manabe, 2016) when citizens gathered to protest the use of nuclear energy and the proposed changes to the Japanese security laws. *Abe yamero* (quit/resign Abe) in particular, was part of a rap-style call-and-response which the youth group Student Emergency Action for Liberal Democracy (SEALDs) performed. The incivility of the imperative, and the five-mora pattern combine to make a distinctive chant. The security laws were passed, and Abe was voted in to a further term in office during which the successful bid to host the 2020 Games was made. Abe resigned in August 2020 due to health reasons leaving behind a long trail of scandals and unresolved disputes. The hashtag *#Abeyamero* circulated on social media for the duration of his term. The hashtag *#Bachkaere* mimics the earlier hashtag not only in linguistic structure (the imperative), but also as metonymy. Prefaced by the last name of an individual, the named individual is foregrounded as not only responsible for, but representative of the injustices and devasting impacts which are the focus of the protest.

The in/civility of the hashtag *#Bachkaere* reimagines the host of the 2020 Games, at the level of the individual. It is no longer the nation, or the Tokyo metropolis which is being asked to bear the burden of the Olympics during the disruptions of the pandemic, but individual people who are affected by a public health crisis. When shared by individuals via social media and in street protests, in/hospitality emerges as a collective act against the demands the Games continue on without regard for the safety of residents of the host city and nation. The frame of polite *omotenashi* which was used to brand the nation within contemporary global geopolitics, is undone by the anti-Olympic movement through impolite demands.

Just as the aesthetic labour of *omotenashi* is mediatised in multimodal texts, *#bachkaere* is utilised in images and actions across the Tokyo metropolis. The citing of the hashtags not only in social media spaces, but also on hand-made placards displayed in the onsite street demonstrations broadcast through online and print media frames the 2020 Games in and of itself as a disruption by accentuating the unwelcomeness of specific guests. The *#Bachkaere* hashtag is one face of dissent performed through protests and demonstrations both online and at sites designed for the Games both inside and outside the Tokyo metropolis. In an increasing networked world connected by a diversity of digital media platforms, connective action emerges.

As the above analysis demonstrates, the framing of the 2020 Games as a "uniquely Japanese" welcoming of visitors is firmly disrupted by the COVID-19 pandemic, and through civil society acts of incivility. Welcoming is reframed as an impossibility by protesters who take a stance against the mega-event proceeding.

6. Un/welcoming "Selfless" Hospitality

The resemiotisation of the term *omotenashi* via multi-layered translatory processes makes recognisable (Butler, 2009) notions of im/politeness on which it pivots. When rendered into English via the notion of "selfless hospitality," the very self who is exerting the "effort" is elided in the ritualistic performance of welcoming. The guest is interpellated into a specific framework of behaviour aimed to showcase the host's performance of "unity" and "diversity" in alliance with the overarching goals of the local and global Olympic movements.

The "polite" *omotenashi* discourse which frames the public campaign at the point of the Bid for the 2020 Games is upended by the beginning of a pandemic which results in postponement of the Games. This postponement intensifies opposition to the Games due to the disruptions the pandemic causes to the everyday life of Tokyoites. The response by civic groups is to interject with "impolite" demands. Regardless of this disruption, in July 2021 as the foreign press, IOC officials and Olympic teams begin to enter Japan for the 2020 Games, the IOC adds the phrase "together" to the official Olympic motto and commences a "Stronger Together" global campaign which strives to recognise "the unifying power of sport and the importance of solidarity." The IOC official website explains that: "The creative campaign celebrates athletes by showcasing their journey to the Olympic Games Tokyo 2020, and how they have kept moving even when the world around them stopped" (July 20, 2021).[4] With residents who are not Japanese nationals still locked out of the country unable to reunite with family or continue to study and/or work, international students and researchers denied passage to Japan, and in the shadow of the death of a migrant held in detention in March 2021, the question of just who is being united by what forms of emotions, and who is being allowed to move forward *together* remains unanswered.

"Hospitality," and "togetherness" are tasked as unifying not only a nation but an international community through the power of sport. Yet they hang precariously as "untranslatable" concepts at a time when borders are closed, and movement is heavily monitored except to a privileged few. In the face of a global pandemic which disrupts a mega-event premised on *omotenashi*, or "selfless hospitality" which leads to "unity in diversity" the event itself flails as everyday citizens are motivated to campaign against excess in unprecedented times. The disruptions result in "impolite" demands which illustrate the impossibility of "selflessness" in a global pandemic which curtails the movement of the public at the expense of global mega-events.

Claire Maree is Professor in Japanese, Asia Institute, University of Melbourne. A queer theorist and linguist, Claire Maree mobilises linguistic and cultural studies methodologies to examine language, identity, and the media. Claire's work has been foundational to the establishment of Japanese language, gender, and sexuality studies.

Notes

[1] The Paralympic Games August 24–September 5, 2021.
[2] Winter Olympics and Paralympics were held in Sapporo in 1972 and Nagano in 1998.
[3] The anti-ANPO demonstrators were protesting against the Treaty of Mutual Cooperation and Security between the USA and Japan, known by the abbreviation 安保 [*anpo*] in Japanese.
[4] https://olympics.com/ioc/olympic-motto.

References

Andersson, Marta. 2021. "The climate of climate change: Impoliteness as a hallmark of homophily in YouTube comment threads on Greta Thunberg's environmental activism." *Journal of Pragmatics* 178 (June): 93–107.

Asahi Shimbun. 2021. "'5th wave' of COVID-19 cases feared in Tokyo and Osaka." July 17, 2021. https://www.asahi.com/ajw/articles/14397380.

Boykoff, Jules. 2014. *Activism and the Olympics: Dissent at the Games in Vancouver and London.* Rutgers University Press.

Boykoff, Jules. 2017. "Protest, activism, and the Olympic Games: An overview of key issues and iconic moments." *International Journal of the History of Sport* 34, no. 3/4: 162–183.

Boykoff, Jules, and Matthew Yasuoka. 2014. "Media coverage of the 2014 Winter Olympics in Sochi, Russia: Putin, politics, and Pussy Riot." *Olympika: The International Journal of Olympic Studies* 23: 27–55.

Butler, Judith. 2009. *Frames of War: When is Life Grievable?* London: Verso.

Collins, Sandra. 2011. "East Asian Olympic desires: Identity on the global stage in the 1964 Tokyo, 1988 Seoul and 2008 Beijing games." *International Journal of the History of Sport* 28, no. 16: 2240–2260.

Davies, Bethan L. Michael Haugh and Andrew John Merrison, eds. 2013. *Situated Politeness.* London: Bloomsbury Academic.

Droubie, Paul. 2011. "Phoenix arisen: Japan as peaceful internationalist at the 1964 Tokyo Summer Olympics." *The International Journal of the History of Sport* 28, no. 16: 2309–2322.

Dunn, Cynthia Dickel. 2006. "Formulaic expressions, Chinese proverbs, and newspaper editorials: Exploring type and token interdiscursivity in Japanese wedding speeches." *Journal of Linguistic Anthropology* 16, no. 2: 153–172. https://doi.org/10.1525/jlin.2006.16.2.153.

Dunn, Cynthia Dickel. 2011. "Formal forms or verbal strategies? Politeness theory and Japanese business etiquette training." *Journal of Pragmatics* 43 no. 15: 3643–3654.

Dunn, Cynthia Dickel. 2018. "Bowing incorrectly: Aesthetic labor and expert knowledge in Japanese business etiquette training." In *Japanese at Work: Politeness, Power, and Personae in Japanese*

Workplace Discourse, edited by Haruko Minegishi Cook and Janet S. Shibamoto-Smith, 15–36. Cham: Springer International Publishing.

Eelen, Gino, 2001. *A Critique of Politeness Theories.* Manchester: St. Jerome.

Girginov, Vassil and Laura Hills. 2008. "A sustainable sports legacy: Creating a link between the London Olympics and sports participation." *The International Journal of the History of Sport* 25, no.14, 2091–2116, https://doi.org/10.1080/09523360802439015.

Giulianotti, Richard, Gary Armstrong, Gavin Hales, and Dick Hobbs. 2015. "Sport mega-events and public opposition: A sociological study of the London 2012 Olympics." *Journal of Sport & Social Issues* 39 no. 2: 99–119.

Goffman, Erving. 1974. *Frame Analysis: An Essay on the Organization of Experience.* Boston: Northeastern University Press.

Haugh, Michael. 2013. "Im/politeness, social practice and the participation order." *Journal of Pragmatics* 58: 52–72.

Holthus, Barbara G., Isaac Gagné, Wolfram Manzenreiter, and Franz Waldenberger, eds. 2020. *Japan through the Lens of the Tokyo Olympics.* New York: Routledge.

Hubbard, Phil and Eleanor Wilkinson 2015. "Welcoming the world? Hospitality, homonationalism, and the London 2012 Olympics." *Antipode* 47, no. 3: 598–615.

Iedema, Rick. 2001. "Resemiotization." *Semiotica* 137, no. 1: 23–39.

Iedema, Rick. 2003. "Multimodality, resemiotization: Extending the analysis of discourse as multi-semiotic practice." *Visual Communication* 2, no. 1: 29–57.

Jackson, Sarah J., and Brooke Foucault Welles. 2015. "Hijacking #Mynypd: Social media dissent and networked counterpublics." *Journal of Communication* 65, no. 6: 932–952.

Jary, Mark. 1998. "Relevance theory and the communication of politeness." *Journal of Pragmatics* 30, no. 1: 1–19.

Manabe, Noriko. 2016. *The Revolution Will Not Be Televised: Protest Music after Fukushima.* New York: Oxford University Press.

McGillivray, David, John Lauermann, and Daniel Turner. 2021. "Event bidding and new media activism." *Leisure Studies* 40, no. 1: 69–81.

Miller, Laura. 2017. "Japan's Trendy Word Grand Prix and Kanji of the Year: Commodified language forms in multiple contexts." In *Language and Materiality: Ethnographic and Theoretical Explorations*, edited by Jillian R. Cavanaugh and Shalini Shankar, 43–62. Cambridge: Cambridge University Press.

Mills, Sara, 2003. *Gender and Politeness.* New York: Cambridge University Press.

Nishimura, Yukiko. 2019. "Impoliteness." In *Routledge Handbook of Japanese Sociolinguistics*, edited by Patrick Heinrich and Yumiko Ohara, 264–278. London: Routledge

No 2020 Olympics Disaster OkotowaLink. 2020. *20 Reasons to Oppose the Tokyo Olympics.*

Ohashi, Jun. 2008. "Linguistic rituals for thanking in Japanese: Balancing obligations." *Journal of Pragmatics* 40, no. 12: 2150–2174.

Olympics.com. 2020. "Framework for the preparation of the Olympic and Paralympic Games following postponement." Accessed August 20, 2021. https://olympics.com/tokyo-2020/en/news/framework-for-the-preparation-of-the-olympic-and-paralympic-games-following-post.

Oostendorp, Marcelyn. 2018. "Extending resemiotisation: Time, space and body in discursive representation." *Social Semiotics* 28, no. 3: 297–314.

Petrovic, Sonja. 2020. "Tracing individual perceptions of media credibility in post-3.11 Japan." *The Asia-Pacific Journal: Japan Focus* 18, no. 10:3. https://apjjf.org/-Sonja-Petrovic/5397/article.pdf.

Pizziconi, Barbara, 2006. "Politeness." In *Encyclopedia of Language & Linguistics*, edited by K. Brown, 679–684. 2nd ed., vol. 9. Oxford: Elsevier.

Pizziconi, Barbara. 2007. "The lexical mapping of politeness in British English and Japanese." *Journal of Politeness Research* 3, no. 2: 207–241.

Reconstruction Agency. n.d. "Recovery Olympics Portal Site." Accessed August 20, 2021. https://www.reconstruction.go.jp/2020portal/eng/.

Takigawa Christel-san kikoku: "Omotenashi" de Gorin shōchi [Ms Christel Takigawa arrives home: "Omotenashi" brings in the Olympic Bid]. *ANN News Channel* (You Tube), September 10, 2013. Accessed August 20, 2021. https://www.youtube.com/watch?v=PCFesHn_GRo.

The Tokyo Organising Committee of the Olympic and Paralympic Games. 2016. *Tokyo 2020 Action & Legacy Plan 2016: Participating in the Tokyo 2020 Games, Connecting with Tomorrow.*

Tokyo 2020 Website. 2013. "Christel Takigawa Joins Tokyo 2020 to Champion Cool Tokyo." 24 June 2013, Tokyo 2020 Website.

Tombleson, Bridget, and Katharina Wolf. 2017. Rethinking the circuit of culture: How participatory culture has transformed cross-cultural communication. *Public Relations Review* 43 no. 1: 14–25. https://doi.org/10.1016/j.pubrev.2016.10.017.

U-can Neologism and Buzzword Award, 2013. Accessed August 20, 2021. https://www.jiyu.co.jp/singo/index.php?eid=00030.

Watts, Richard J. 1992. "Linguistic politeness and politic verbal behaviour: Reconsidering claim for universality". In *Politeness in Language: Studies in its History, Theory and Practice*, edited by Richard J. Watts, Sachiko Ide, Konrad Ehlich, 43–69. Berlin: Mouton de Gruyter.

Xiong, Ying, Moonhee Cho, and Brandon Boatwright. 2019. "Hashtag activism and message frames among social movement organizations: Semantic network analysis and thematic analysis of Twitter during the #MeToo movement." *Public Relations Review* 45, no. 1: 10–23.

Yang, Guobin. 2016. "Narrative agency in hashtag activism: The case of #BlackLivesMatter." *Media and Communication* 4, no. 4: 13–17.

Zappavigna, Michele. 2015. "Searchable talk: The linguistic functions of hashtags." *Social Semiotics* 25. no. 3: 274–291.

CHAPTER 5

Political Leaders' Discourse Addressing "Corona Discrimination" in Japan

Ikuko Nakane

Abstract

This chapter discusses discursive resources and underlying ideological stances of four central and regional government leaders' public video messages to counter widespread "coronavirus discrimination" discourse in Japan. Analysis reveals intersecting layers of discourses which emerge from different socio-political positioning of the creators of the messages. Their messages seek cooperation from the public while aligning themselves with their institutional agenda. The anti-discrimination messages were also characterised by the use of the war metaphor "fight against the virus," whereby corona discrimination is discursively projected as disruption to the national unity required in a public health crisis. The counter-discourse to highly disruptive discourse of discrimination by the leaders implicitly addresses potential loss of political power and control.

Keywords: anti-discrimination, video message, political leaders, metaphor, institutional discourse

1. Introduction

When Japan was hit by the triple disaster of 2011, a strong sense of solidarity emerged from the national recovery effort. However, as the nation faced the COVID-19 pandemic in 2020, disturbing instances of discrimination against people who contracted the virus, health workers, essential workers and their families were reported. Media reports of コロナ差別 [*korona sabetsu*] (lit. corona discrimination) revealed examples such as recovered patients being told not to come to work and hospital employees being asked not to bring their children to childcare. A database search brought up the earliest articles with the terms コロナ [*korona*] and 差別 [*sabetsu*] in *Yomiuri Shimbun* published on January 31, 2020 (*Yomiuri Shimbun*, 2020a), and in *Asahi Shimbun* (*Asahi Shimbun*, 2020a) on February 1, 2020. The target expanded from Chinese people to Japanese citizens returning from China, and to doctors who treated patients who contracted the disease on the cruise ship

Diamond Princess. As community transmission began to spread in Japan, those who caught the illness, essential workers such as doctors, nurses, truck drivers, their families, and even visitors/outsiders from other prefectures became the target. Even drivers of cars with non-local registrations were told to leave and sent back to their own region. This corona discrimination began to cause noticeable disruptions to the medical, economic, and social welfare of the nation. Thus, an urgent need to put this "disruptive discourse" under control emerged.

Reacting to this, human rights organisations, the Japanese Red Cross Society and grassroots community groups launched advocacy campaigns. The government had to act on the discrimination as a social and public health problem, and so drew up a policy in response to COVID-19 and implemented the Act on Special Measures for Pandemic Influenza and New Infectious Diseases Preparedness and Response (implemented on March 14, 2020). Government departments, prefectural governments, and municipal councils have also taken some measures by sending messages to the general public, and in some prefectures and councils, ordinances have been implemented to forbid "unjust discrimination" and "slander" in relation to COVID-19.

In times of health crisis, community leaders have responsibility and power to send messages to the public, as they "have credibility because they can say and do what is necessary to protect the lives and livelihoods of the publics" (Littlefield, 2021, p. 369). Leaders' messages are also important because of the impact of human behaviour on the spread of an infectious disease (O'Hair and O'Hair, 2021). Since the COVID-19 pandemic began, leaders around the world have been sending messages to the public using various modes of communication in their effort to address the public health crisis. A number of recent studies examined leaders' communication strategies (e.g., Reyes Bernard et al., 2021; Dada et al., 2021; Littlefield, 2021; Manfredi-Sánchez et al., 2021) and identified their leadership stances. Since "the way health messages are framed and communicated has a profound impact on public trust and compliance with public health measures" (Dada et al., 2021, p. 1), it is worth closely examining the discourse of leaders' public messages.

Stigma and discrimination associated with COVID-19 are detrimental not only to the effort to stop the spread of the virus but also to humanity (World Health Organization, n.d.). Given the extent of corona discrimination reported in Japan, which has led to official regulations to counter it (albeit non-punitive), political leaders had to address the public in their constituencies directly. How did community leaders, who assume the authority and power to send a strong message to the public, address COVID-19-related discrimination in their public discourse in Japan? This chapter explores how policy-makers utilised discursive resources in their video messages to persuade the public to stop corona discrimination.

2. The Video Messages

The video messages of two central government ministers and two prefectural governors were analysed for this chapter. Aside from these four politicians, many leaders of prefectures and local councils published similar messages online, but the selection was made as the two government ministers had specifically relevant roles (one in charge of COVID-19 measures, another in charge of the justice ministry, which addresses human rights issues), and the Tokyo and Osaka governors were the most visible figures in Japan's regional politics. The two groups of politicians, from central government and regional government, were selected as the latter could draw on "closeness" to the audience owing to regional affiliation. The following video messages from two central government ministers and two prefectural governors were selected for this chapter:

1. Minister in charge of Novel Coronavirus Yasutoshi Nishimura (September 4, 2020, 2 minutes 20 seconds)
偏見・差別に対するメッセージ [*Henken, sabetsu ni taisuru messēji*] (Message against prejudice and discrimination)
Office of Novel Coronavirus Disease Control, Cabinet Secretariat YouTube channel
https://www.youtube.com/watch?v=vvF3fJsFdcA
2. Justice Minister Masako Mori (May 1, 2020, 3 minutes)
新型コロナウィルス感染症に関連した差別や虐待に対する法務大臣ビデオメッセージ [*Shingata korona uirusu kansenshō ni kanrenshita sabetsu ya gyakutai ni taisuru hōmudaijin bideo messēji*] (Justice minister's video message on discrimination and abuse associated with novel coronavirus disease]
Ministry of Justice YouTube channel
https://www.youtube.com/watch?v=RYSooqCxo-o
3. Tokyo Governor Yuriko Koike (22 June, 2020, 1 minute 14 seconds)
ストップ！コロナ差別小池百合子東京都知事からのメッセージ [*STOP! Korona sabetsu: Koike Yuriko Tokyo Tochiji kara no messēji*] (STOP! Corona discrimination: A message from Tokyo Governor Yuriko Koike)
Tokyo Metropolitan Government official YouTube channel
https://www.youtube.com/watch?v=KyPwDBKz920
4. Osaka Governor Hirofumi Yoshimura (July 1, 2020, 2 minutes 13 seconds)
ストップ！コロナ差別吉村大阪府知事からのメッセージ [*STOP! Korona sabetsu: Yoshimura Ōsaka Fuchiji kara no messēji*] (STOP! Corona discrimination: A message from Osaka Governor Yoshimura)
Osaka Prefectural Government official YouTube channel
https://www.youtube.com/watch?v=bobLDEjiXtM

Transcripts were made of the video messages, and other semiotic resources in the videos such as the background, words, and names appearing in the video were analysed, together comprising a discourse-semiotic "package."

3. Analytical Approaches

The analysis in this chapter is informed by Systemic Functional Linguistics (SFL) (Halliday, 1985) and Critical Discourse Analysis (CDA) (van Dijk, 1993a). In Halliday's (1985) view, language serves to make meanings as social semiotics, and those meanings have three domains: ideational, interpersonal, and textual. Ideational meanings concern our experiences in the world realised through the system of transitivity, interpersonal meanings concern the nature of exchange carried out through language and the tenor of the discourse associated with the relationship between the participants (realised through the system of mood and modality), and textual meanings concern how semiotic resources in the discourse are bound together as a coherent and cohesive whole through the structure of theme and rheme. Theme is "the point of departure for the message" and "that with which the clause is concerned," and rheme is "the part in which the theme is developed" (Halliday, 1985, p. 38). The discourse data were analysed by focusing on what types of experiences (or processes), exchanges (actions), and themes were presented.

Critical Discourse Analysis complements the Hallidayan approach to discourse by bringing wider sociocultural, historical, and political perspectives into the analysis. It focuses on how language at different levels—for example pronouns, lexical items, turn-taking, and narrative structures—contributes to reproducing or challenging the power and dominance of groups and people in authority (van Dijk, 1993a). While CDA has contributed to revealing how racism or other forms of discrimination are legitimised through political discourse, for example elite racism (van Dijk, 1993b), the present chapter focuses on how the Japanese politicians offer their *counter*-discrimination discourse. CDA offers opportunities for revealing institutional and political agendas layered onto the multimodal video discourse data. In the development of CDA, the important role of visual elements in multimodal texts has also been recognised as one of the key communication strategies for manipulating ideologies (van Dijk, 2006). The focus on the role of multimodal discourse from the CDA perspective as a vehicle to mediate, promote, and challenge ideologies enables us to scrutinise the leaders' socio-political agenda (not limited to their urgent need to bring the disruption of social cohesion under control) in their messages. The approach to multimodal analysis informed by the principles of SFL and developed by Kress and van Leeuwen (2021) is widely adopted in studies of public and media discourse, and this chapter will be informed by the same approach. In particular, I draw on its principles of "composition" whereby each element of a multimodal text itself realises layered meanings but also comes together with other elements to create meanings as a whole (ibid.).

4. Analysis of the Video Messages

4.1 Stances in Presenting the Problem

In all four video messages, corona discrimination is foregrounded as the topical theme, and presented as a phenomenon which "exists," or is "spreading."

1. Minister Nishimura

エッセンシャルワーカーの方々、こうした方々やそのご家族、関係者に対する謂れのない偏見・差別が残念ながら存在しています。

[*Essensharuwākā no katagata, kōshita katagata ya sono gokazoku, kankeisha ni taisuru iwarenonai henken, sabetsu ga zannennagara **sonzaishite imasu**.*]

"There **exists** unfounded prejudice and discrimination against essential workers, those workers and their families, associates."

2. Governor Koike

今、新型コロナウィルス感染症に感染された方やそのご家族に対する心無い書き込みがSNSなどで広がっています。

[*Ima, shingata koronauirusu kansenshō ni kansensareta kata ya sono gokazoku ni taisuru kokoronai kakikomi ga SNS nado de **hirogatte imasu**.*]

(Currently, hurtful posts about people who contracted novel coronavirus and their family members **are spreading** in places like SNS.)

Three of the videos (Nishimura, Mori, Koike) contain a statement denouncing corona discrimination. In terms of modality, these statements contain adverbs of degree or usuality (cf. Halliday, 1985, p. 82) such as "*zettaini*" (absolutely/never) and "*kesshite*" (never) to send a strong message to the public.

3. Minister Nishimura

このような行為は絶対に許されません。

[*Konoyōna kōi wa **zettaini** yurusaremasen.*]

(Such actions are **never** tolerated.)

4. Minister Mori

こうした方々を傷つけるような不当な差別や偏見は決してあってはなりません。

[*Kōshita katagata o kizutukeru yōna futōna sabetsu ya henken wa **kesshite** atte wa narimasen.*]

(Unjust discrimination and prejudice, which hurt these people, should **never** take place.)

5. Governor Koike

こうした不当な差別・偏見や誹謗中傷は決して許されるものではありません。

[*Kōshita futōna sabetsu, henken ya hibō chūshō wa **kesshite** yurusareru mono dewa arimasen.*]

(Such unjust discrimination, prejudice and abuse are **never** to be tolerated.)

Unlike the three leaders above, Osaka Governor Yoshimura introduces the topic of corona discrimination while flagging the purpose of the video message. Utilising a *no-wa* cleft sentence structure, whose key function in oral presentation is anticipatory (Kaneyasu, 2019, p. 18), he flags the point of his message early on.

6. Governor Yoshimura

合わせて皆さんにお願いしたいのは、このコロナによる差別、これを是非なくしていただきたいということです。

[*Awasete **minasan ni onegaishitai** no wa, kono korona ni yoru sabetsu, kore o **zehi**, **nakushite itadakitai** toiu koto desu.*]

(Also, what **[I] would like to ask you** to do, is that **[I] would like you to eliminate** this corona-based discrimination, **by all means**.)

While it is a declarative sentence, a request is embedded with an emphasis for obligation *zehi* (by all means). Yoshimura's framing of the presentation of the problem serves as a pointer to the overall aim of the message. A statement with "discrimination" as a subject/topic follows the above statement:

7. Governor Yoshimura

ウィルスの恐怖はそのウィルスそのものの恐怖だけではなくて、それによる差別、それによる社会の分断、そういったことによる恐怖、これも実は非常に我々としては避けなければならないことだという風に思います。

[*Uirusu no kyōfu wa sono uirusu sonomono no kyōfu dake dewa nakute, sore ni yoru **sabetsu**, sore ni yoru shakai no bundan, sōitta koto niyoru kyōfu, kore mo jitsu wa hijōni **wareware** toshite wa sakenakereba naranai koto da toiu fūni **omoimasu**.*]

(The fear of the virus is not the fear of the virus itself, but **discrimination** because of it, and social divisions because of it, fear because of these things, this is actually something **we** really have to avoid, **[I] think**.)

This statement sets the message apart from the other three video messages because of the participants, or agents, it contains. First, "we" (*wareware*), as an assumed actor of discrimination, and "[I] think" (*omoimasu*—"I" is assumed in this context) as the owner of this message. Yoshimura's message places him and the general public as participants in the problem of corona discrimination. In the other leaders' statements (1)–(5) above, victims of discrimination are mentioned but not the general public (audience) or the speaker's own mental process.

4.2 Interpersonal Concerns in Requesting Co-operation

In order to contain the disease, the leaders' messages need to mobilise people's cooperation. This involves asking the public to counter corona discrimination, which concerns interpersonal meaning and calls for analysis of speech act and modality (cf. Halliday, 1985). Towards the end of all the video messages, imperative structures demanding action appear, with various modal expressions.

Below, the minister in charge of COVID-19 Yasutoshi Nishimura makes requests using a neutrally polite form "*onegaishimasu*" ([I] would like to request), but also with an imperative structure with a respectful honorific expression "*gokakuninkudasai*" (Please check). He ends his message with "[I] would like to ask for your cooperation," this time with a humble honorific request "*onegaiitashimasu*" ([I] would like to request), accompanied by a bow.

8. Minister Nishimura

まず、差別的な言動には同調せず、理性的な判断をお願いします。CORONA.GO.JPなど信頼できる機関からの正確な情報をご確認ください。みなさんのご協力をよろしくお願いいたします。

[*Mazu, sabetsutekina gendō ni wa dōchōsezu, riseitekina handan o* **onegaishimasu**. *CORONA.GO.JP nado shinraidekiru kikan kara no seikakuna jōhō o* **gokakuninkudasai**. *Minasan no gokyōryoku o yoroshiku* **onegaiitashimasu**.]

(First, **[I] would like to request** [you] not go along with discriminatory language and behaviour but instead use rational judgement. **Please check** accurate information from reliable organizations such as corona.go.jp. Your cooperation **would be** greatly **appreciated**.)

Minister Nishimura's language is formal and respectful towards the audience. Tokyo Governor Yuriko Koike, as we can see below, also uses an imperative structure but with a polite volitional form for invitation "*mashō*" (Let's), whereby she invites the audience to thank the essential workers and send their support to them. This invitation is accompanied by an emphatic nod and open arms. In this way, she attempts to mobilise the community with a collective positive action. The invitation also contains a polite humble honorific lexis "*mairu*" (go) (*okutte mairimashō* "let's send on"), and the contribution of the essential workers is also expressed with an honorific "*sasaete kudasaru*" (instead of the neutral *kureru*), together showing respect towards health and essential workers. Both Nishimura and Koike are respectful to the audience, but these honorific expressions also demonstrate elegance and sophistication (cf. Dunn, 2013).

9. Governor Koike

こうした私たちの生活基盤を支えてくださるエッセンシャルワーカーの皆さんに感謝すると共に、エール
を送ってまいりましょう。

[*Kōshita watashitachi no sēkatsukiban o sasaete kudasaru essensharuwākā no minasama ni kanshasuru to tomoni, ēru o okutte **mairimashō**.*]

(Let us thank these essential workers who provide support for our livelihoods, and send them our cheers.)

Osaka Governor Yoshimura's message also contains a *mashō* invitation: "*Korona niyoru sabetsu, kore wa zettaini nakushite ikimashō.*" (Discrimination based on corona, let's definitely eliminate it.) However, he does not use an honorific *mairu* (go) as in Koike's message (9) above, but the neutral verb *iku* (go). Yoshimura is more than twenty years Koike's junior and has gained strong popularity in the prefecture where his supporters seem to find his refreshing and direct youthfulness appealing (Kimura, 2021). The two governors seem to be using different interpersonal discourse strategies to appeal to their support bases.

In (10) below, Yoshimura actually uses a humble honorific form of an auxiliary verb *itadaku* (to have something done), in other requests to the public. However, in "*yameteitadakitai*" ([I] would like you to stop, lit. [I] want you to kindly stop), he uses the verb "*yameru*" (stop) and a combination of auxiliary "*-tai*" ([I] want to), addressing the audience more directly than other politicians. The other leaders presented the core of the anti-discrimination message in a declarative structure which had the role of giving information, as in excerpts (3), (4), and (5) above. Yoshimura's request is also repeated, with the addition of a modal adverb *zettaini* (definitely), making the demand more forceful. At the same time, both requests end with "*to omoimasu*" ([I] think), which mitigates the imposition as a mood adjunct (Eggins, 1994, p. 182) but also brings a personal touch. This solidarity-oriented approach may have more appeal to the audience. According to a survey conducted by *Asahi Shimbun* (*Asahi Shimbun*, 2020b), Governor Yoshimura rose to the top as a politician whose response to the pandemic was evaluated highly by the public, followed by Tokyo Governor Koike.

10. Governor Yoshimura

特に、感染された方や医療従事者の方への差別はやめていただきたいと思います。[…] そういった方
々への差別というのは、絶対にやめていただきたいと思います。

[*Tokuni, kansensareta kata ya iryōjūjisha no kata e no sabetsu wa, **yameteitadakitai** to omoimasu.* [...] *sōitta katagata e no sabetsu toiu no wa, zettaini **yameteitadakitai** to omoimasu.*]

(In particular, **[I] would like [you] to stop** discrimination against people who contracted the virus and health workers. [...] **[I] would like [you] to stop discriminating against those people at any cost.**)

Yoshimura's requests above with the verb *"yameru"* are in fact cohesive with his final utterance in the video, which is also the title of the video message: "STOP! Corona discrimination." The imperative sentence STOP! コロナ差別 is a bilingual slogan, with "STOP!" written in English and *"Korona sabetsu"* written in a combination of katakana and kanji. It is interesting that this slogan is also used at the end of, and as the title of, Tokyo Governor Koike's message. The slogan originates in the Centre for Human Rights Education and Training's campaign "STOP! コロナ差別―差別をなくし正しい理解を―キャンペーン" [*Sutoppu! Korona sabetsu — sabetsu o nakushi tadashī rikai o — kyanpēn*] (STOP! Corona discrimination campaign: Eliminate discrimination and have a correct understanding) (translation by the author) launched on May 17, 2020 (CHRET, 2020). It is now almost ubiquitously adopted by the central and prefectural governments, as well as municipalities across Japan, although in some cases the English word "stop" is replaced with its Japanese equivalent *"yameyō"* (let's stop). It is worth noting that the most direct way to demand the required action from the public is realised in English in those governors' messages, especially given a set of katakana characters（ストップ）is available to represent English loanwords in Japanese, in addition to the Japanese *"yameyō."* We see an example of "salience" (Kress and van Leeuwen, 2021, p. 210) doing meaning-making work through the choice of typography and code. Koike pronounces the word more like a loanword, with the final [p] sound followed by [u] while Yoshimura's ended with [p], but as Seargeant (2011) states, "the boundary between 'English' and 'Japanese' is nebulous" (p. 199), especially where the word is used as part of a slogan but not as a lingua franca (cf. Seargeant, 2011). Given that "STOP! Corona discrimination" is a campaign slogan, the interpersonal impact of this direct command with a word borrowed from English and written in Roman alphabet (in the title and subtitles in the video) may not be as significant as the indirect imperatives used in the governors' messages. Furthermore, the English word "stop" allows for two interpretations of this slogan, which the Japanese word *"yameru"* cannot provide: one should stop discrimination against others, or stop others' acts of discrimination. The choice of the lexis and script on one hand seems to make the campaign visible and effective, but on the other serves to mitigate the force of the message, for fear of losing support from the audience.

4.3 Legitimising the Government in Action

The leaders present messages as representatives of the government or the ministry, and their videos also serve to legitimise these organisations' actions and image. Their discourse structures and strategies serve to enact and reproduce their preferred ideologies, which favours authorities in power (van Dijk, 1993a). To enhance the image of a particular group, discourse strategies can be used to promote ideologies of "us" versus "them," emphasising "good 'properties/actions' of 'us' while emphasising 'bad properties/actions' of 'them'" (van Dijk, 1998, p. 33). The use of referent terms and their "actions" and "properties" in parts of the video messages suggests that such discourse strategies were adopted in the videos examined in this chapter.

Justice Minister Mori's message is distinctive from the other leaders' in that it targets both the audience and victims, with more focus on the latter. The video message is accessed via the link provided on the page "Measures taken by the Ministry of Justice to eliminate corona discrimination" (Ministry of Justice, n.d., translation by the author), which is one of the MoJ Human Rights Bureau sites. The message addresses corona discrimination as a human rights issue, and at the beginning of the video, the minister is introduced by human rights image mascot characters *Jinken mamoru kun* and *Jinken ayumi chan* (lit. "Human rights protection" and "Human rights step forward," but *mamoru* and *ayumi* are also common Japanese given names), designed by a well-known cartoonist. These mascots sit on either side of the minister with open arms while the message is delivered, reinforcing the human rights stance of the minister's message from the margins (Kress and van Leeuwen, 2021, p. 210), yet at the same time making the disturbing nature of the issue at hand accessible with their cuteness.

The human rights angle is highlighted not only by the semiotic resources above, but also in the interpersonal moves in Mori's discourse. In her message, she first thanks the general public, who have been cooperating with the restrictions, and then the health workers and other essential workers, with abundant use of honorifics. After condemning corona discrimination (see Excerpt [4] above), the minister states that the Human Rights Bureau has a helpline for people:

11. Minister Mori

私たちは、みなさんの助けになりたいと考えています。法務省の人権擁護機関では、差別や虐待などのさまざまな事件問題について、電話やインターネットで相談を受け付けています。

[*Watashitachi wa, minasan no tasuke ni naritai to kangaeteimasu. Hōmushō no jinkenyōgo kikan dewa, sabetsu ya gyakutai nado no samazamana jinken mondai nitsuite, denwa ya intānetto de sōdan o uketsuketeimasu.*]

(We would like to help you. The Human Rights Bureau of the Ministry of Justice has telephone and internet consultation services for various human rights issues such as discrimination and abuse.)

This is when personal pronouns signal a shift in participant roles and the addressivity, where "we"—the MoJ Human Rights Bureau—is foregrounded in the discourse, and the addressee(s) "you" are the victim(s) of corona discrimination. The imperative structure *kudasai* (please [action]) appears in all of the last six sentences, encouraging victims to reach out to the bureau via its hotline, with Mori's final message " 一人で悩まずにどうぞご相談ください" [*Hitori de nayamazu ni dōzo, gosōdan kudasai*] (Instead of suffering on your own, **please** reach out to us.). The moves and themes in Mori's message underscore the MoJ's stance that its main role is to protect the human rights of the victims by offering them support. The video, including the non-verbal semiotic resources, thus also signals the ministry is doing its job, thus legitimising its authority and role in government.

The "government in action" is also foregrounded in the message of the minister in charge of COVID-19 Nishimura. Unlike Minister Mori, he directs the message at the general public and requests their cooperation in addressing the discrimination, but also informs the audience what the government is doing to address "this issue":

12. Minister Nishimura

政府として、この問題に対応していくため、各分野の専門家と省庁横断によるワーキンググループを発足させ、9月1日に第一回会合を開催しました。… 感染拡大を防止していくための課題や対応策について具体的な議論を行っていきます。

[*Sēfu toshite, kono mondai ni taiōshite iku tame, kaku bunya no senmonka to shōchō ōdan niyoru wākingugurūpu o hossokusase, kugatsu tuitachi ni **daiikkai kaigō o kai-saiitashimashita**. … kansen kakudai o bōshi shiteiku tameno kadai ya taiōsaku nitsuite **gutaitekina giron o okonatte ikimasu**.*]

(To address this problem, **the government has launched** a cross-ministry **working group** with experts from various fields, and **held the first meeting** on the 1st of September. … [We] **will have concrete discussions** on issues and measures in relation to preventing the spread of infections.)

The processes realised in the clauses in the above excerpt are the government's actions such as "*taiōshiteiku*" (deal with), "*hossokusase*" (launched), "*kaisaiitashimashita*" (held), and "*giron o okonatteikimasu*" (will have discussions). Nishimura highlights the fact that the government is taking actions, and then asks the public to avoid going along with discriminatory behaviour and seek information from a reliable source (see Excerpt [8] above). Thus, the minister presents a positive picture of the government in action, while justifying the requests made to the public.

These two government ministers also had their governmental roles "Minister in charge of Novel Coronavirus" and "Minister of Justice" displayed in the video. Nishimura's role was also accompanied by the emblem of the Cabinet Secretariat, and Mori spoke in front of a panel with 法務省 [*Hōmushō*] (Ministry of Justice) and its emblem "MoJ." This use of semiotic resources foregrounds the institutional identities of the ministers positioned at the centre of the screen as representatives of relevant government sections, and the messages also inform the audience that the government is doing its job.

The governors' videos do not show any emblems, their names, or their own professional roles. They sit in front of a plain office wall and introduce themselves as the governor of the region. The only noticeable visual semiotic resource is the Osaka governor's polo shirt, with the logo of EXPO 2025, which Osaka is hosting. Yoshimura is also known for his effort to shift the concentration of power from Tokyo and promote Osaka as another capital of Japan. His video message also contains a specific reference to Osaka managing to "suppress the first wave (of infections) thanks to your understanding and cooperation." Thus, with the Osaka EXPO brand, an image of a successful leader is presented. It is interesting that Koike's message does not explicitly convey the image of "government in action" nor is it scaffolded by non-verbal visual resources. The effort to enhance institutional or leadership visibility may not have been necessary given her well-established profile as a politician and former journalist.

4.4 The 'War' Metaphor for Uniting the Community

Metaphors can be effective rhetorical strategies to advance certain types of ideological stances through discourse and impact on social attitudes (van Dijk, 1993a). Three of the leaders in this study adopted a metaphor associated with "war," some using the word *tatakau*, using the analogy of "fighting" against the virus. Metaphors associated with "war" are not unique to Japanese in public discourse on COVID-19, or unique to discourse on COVID-19 itself (Chung, 2011, Dada et al., 2021). In their discussion of political leaders' speeches during the COVID-19 pandemic, Dada et al. (2021) report that 17 out of 20 heads of government around the world used metaphors associated with "war" (p. 7). Molnár, Takács, and Harnos (2021) specifically examined war and military metaphors in public discourse of the Hungarian prime minister and found that these metaphors helped justify emergency measures and promote national unity. It is worth looking closely at how this metaphor is used by Japanese politicians in addressing the specific issue of discrimination based on COVID-19.

The use of the "fight" metaphor involves two actors in the video messages: health workers and the nation/society. The two governors remind the audience that discriminating against health workers, who are protecting them, is wrong. The following comment from Governor Yoshimura comes after his request to stop the discrimination against infected people and health workers:

13. Governor Yoshimura

医療従事者の方は自分の危険と引き換えにこのコロナと闘う、命を守ってくれてる皆さんです。

[*Iryōjūjisha no kata wa jibun no kiken to hikikae ni kono **korona to tatakau**, inochi o mamottekureteru minasan desu.*]

(Health workers are the people who **fight against corona** at their own risk, and are protecting our lives.)

The adverbial phrase "at their own risk" reinforces the sense of emergency, and "*inochi o mamottekureteru*" (protecting our lives) with its donatory auxiliary verb *kureru* (receiving a favour) implies that we should be more grateful towards health workers. Tokyo Governor Koike also expresses her appreciation towards hard-working health workers who "are fighting so hard," again using the donatory auxiliary *kureru* (in its honorific form *kudasaru*, again being more polite than her Osaka counterpart), while using the phrase *iwarenonai* (unjust) to condemn discrimination against them. The term *kenmei ni* literally means "for dear life," again reinforcing the danger in the "fight against the virus":

14. Governor Koike
また、医療現場の最前線で懸命に闘ってくださっている医療関係者やそのお子さんが謂れのない差別に苦しむ事例も発生しています。
[*Mata, iryōgenba no saizenzen de kenmei ni **tatakatte kudasatteiru** iryō kankeisha ya sono okosan ga **iwarenonai sabetsu** ni kurushimu jirei mo hasseishiteimasu.*]
(Also, there are cases where health workers, who **are fighting** so hard at the frontline of medical institutions, and their children are suffering from **unjust discrimination**.)

The actors of the fight against the virus in the two governors' messages are also the general public, as we can see below:

15. Governor Yoshimura
コロナに打ち勝つ社会を作っていくためには、医学的な知識や、我々行政の力だけではできません。
[*Korona ni **uchikatsu shakai** o tsukutte iku tame ni wa, igakuteki na chishiki ya, wareware gyōsei no chikara dake de wa dekimasen.*]
(To create a **society** that **beats** corona, medical knowledge and the government's power are not enough.)
16. Governor Koike
戦うべき本当の相手はウィルスです。
[*Tatakau beki hontō no aite wa uirusu desu.*]
(The real opponent [we] **should fight against** is the virus.)

It is worth noting that Yoshimura earlier in his message says "social divisions caused by fear of the virus" should be avoided (see [7] above), foregrounding the importance of a social unity which does not tolerate discrimination. Tokyo Governor Koike's message also attempts to mobilise the people by using a "war" metaphor, with the word *tatakau* (fight) here paired with a modal expression of obligation *beki* (should), which sends a strong message to the audience. The phrase "the real opponent" here implies that people should *not* be fighting against other people. The sentence does not have the actor for the verb *takakau* (fight), but "we" is assumed here as the predicate of the preceding sentence contains *mashō* (let's) (see [9] above). Interestingly, Koike's message in (16) above shares some features with one of the key messages in the campaign against corona discrimination by Centre for Human Rights Education and Training (CHRET) about a month earlier: "*Osoreru beki wa hito de wa naku uirusu desu*" (What we should fear is not people but the virus) (CHRET, 2020). The references to "fear" (verb *osoreru* and noun *kyōfu*) are also made in the Japanese Red Cross Society's campaign against discrimination and prejudice, where *kyōfu* (fear) is presented as the root of the problem (Japanese Red Cross Society, 2020).

CHRET's website for the campaign against corona discrimination contains links to video messages of more than twenty prominent community figures. One is from Tsuyoshi Kitazawa, a former football player and currently a sport commentator, who used the fight metaphor in "*Tatakau aite wa korona desu. Hito dewa arimasen.*" (The opponent is corona. Not people). Tokyo Governor Koike's statement in (16) above, which adopts the structure "... *beki*... *wa* ... *desu*" (What [we] should ... is ...) with the "fight" metaphor, has since become the centrepiece of the Tokyo Metropolitan Government's campaign flyer. This flyer also contains the final slogan in Koike's video message: "STOP! Corona discrimination" (CHRET permits the use of its campaign logo and slogans to spread the message). Koike is well known for her creative use of slogans, which seems to have been applied to her anti-discrimination message too.

The two governors draw on this "fight" metaphor, creating a narrative highlighting the importance of social unity. The united front against the virus is also encouraged by use of a war metaphor in Justice Minister Mori's message:

17. Minister Mori
国民が一丸となって感染の拡大に立ち向かうべき時にこうした方々を傷つけるような不当な差別や偏見は決してあってはなりません。

[*Kokumin ga ichigan to natte kansen no kakudai ni tachimukau beki toki ni kōshita katagata o kizutsukeru yōna futōna sabetsu ya henken wa kesshite atte wa narimasen.*]

(When the citizens are obligated to **take a united stand against** the spread of infections, unfair discrimination and prejudice that hurts those people should never take place.)

Along with the expression "*tachimukau*" (stand against), the modal of obligation "*beki*" is used here again, sending a strong message to the public that it is time to unite (*ichigan to natte*). The examples above point to the appeal of war metaphors as an effective rhetorical strategy not only for enhancing compliance with public health measures but also for addressing division in society (which in turn strengthens collective disease prevention).

5. Discussion

The goal of these politicians was to address the same discrimination issue, raise awareness, and shift the public's behaviour. While the leaders adopt similar strategies to achieve their goals, there are also differences in their approaches to appealing to the public. In terms of message content, leaders unequivocally and strongly denounce corona discrimination, but in the manner of delivery, Osaka Governor Yoshimura takes a different stance with a more direct and personal request to the public than the others, whose statements obscure the agency of discriminatory actions (for example, "Discrimination should never be tolerated"). The positioning of the leaders is also varied. Minister Nishimura, who is specifically in charge of COVID-19 in the central government, presents himself in a more explicitly institutional framing, highlighting the actions the government is taking, and directing the public specifically to the government website on COVID-19. Minister Mori, also positioning herself fully in her justice ministry portfolio verbally and non-verbally, focuses on human rights and reaches out to the victims. It is noteworthy that the two government ministers use the request form (*"kudasai"*) to ask the victims to use the ministry's human rights hotline, and to ask the public to refer to the government's own website, while obscuring the person responsible for discrimination. Governor Koike's message also condemns corona discrimination without a participant, but her polite invitation to support essential workers includes herself in the expected action, while utilising strongly worded slogans to mobilise the public to "fight against the virus" and "stop corona discrimination."

It is important to recognise intertextual contexts of the leaders' messages, as there are other public campaigns addressing corona discrimination. As mentioned earlier, some of the key concepts and discursive resources are also found in advocacy campaigns of the Japanese Red Cross Society and CHRET. In order to enhance the effectiveness of the message for the "fight" against the coronavirus, slogans such as "stop corona discrimination" and the metaphor of war travelled across the genres and domains and circulated in public discourse. Blommaert (2005) suggests that in the process of decontextualisation and recontextualisation, "all kinds of mappings are performed, often deeply different from the ones performed in the initial act of communication" (p. 76). While CHRET's "STOP! Corona discrimination" slogan is adopted across the nation as it is, one of the slogans for the CHRET campaign "What we should fear is not people but the virus" (CHRET, 2020), as shown earlier, shares some features with the Tokyo Metropolitan Government's campaign slogan "The real opponent we should fight against is the virus," included in the governor's video message. While CHRET's campaign is oriented to the issue of human rights violation itself, the adoption of the war metaphor (fight) in the leader's message creates a new context where corona discrimination is an obstacle to uniting the people in the face of a public health crisis (cf. Dada et al., 2021).

The absurdity of discriminating against essential workers despite their invaluable contributions in a "fight" against the virus is touched upon by all four leaders. Editorials of major newspapers such as *Asahi Shimbun* and *Yomiuri Shimbun* have also detailed discrimination against essential workers and people who contracted the virus, and the public health consequences of such heinous acts. *Yomiuri Shimbun* (2020b), for example, urged people to act calmly "based on accurate information" in its April 23 editorial, which both Minister Nishimura and Governor Koike emphasise in their videos. Governor Koike's message is also aligned with editorials which encourage people to offer support and express thanks to essential workers (see Excerpt [9] above). For example, the April 19 *Asahi* editorial states "今は拍手を送って感謝と支援の思いを伝える時だ" [*Ima wa hakushu o okutte kansha to shien no omoi o tsutaeru toki da*] (Now is the time to applaud them and express our thanks and support) (*Asahi Shimbun*, 2020c).

It should be noted that these *Asahi* and *Yomiuri* editorial opinions also share messages promoted by other organisations such as the Japanese Red Cross Society. Thus, some aspects of anti-discrimination campaign texts are circulating across public discourses, and in their recontextualisation process, they are mapped out to align with individual message senders' multifaceted agendas. Sometimes, such intertextual relations may also be explicit and deliberate, as we can see in the April 19 *Asahi Shimbun* editorial:

> 18. *Asahi Shimbun* editorial (April 19, 2020)
> 首相や各知事から改めて強いメッセージを発して、社会に呼びかけてほしい。
> [*Shushō ya kaku chiji kara aratamete tsuyoi messēji o hasshite, shakaini yobikakete hoshii.*]
> (We hope that the prime minister and governors send strong messages, and appeal to the community.)

In the above sentence, the editorial directly appeals to the nation's leaders to act on the problem. In his analysis of Japanese newspaper editorials (including *Asahi* and *Yomiuri*), Nanri (2005) finds that "Japanese newspapers tend to leave the solution of the issue under discussion with a large political system" (p. 185). It seems that this is what the *Asahi* editorial is doing, and the leaders have taken up the plea. What is interesting, though, is that the leaders are generally focused on the immediate fight against the virus, while the editorials mentioned above treat corona discrimination as a social issue in the wider socio-historical context of Japan. The title of the *Asahi* editorial is "コロナと差別:社会の荒廃を防ぐため" [*Korona to sabetsu: Shakai no kōhai o fusegu tame*] (Corona and discrimination: To avoid dilapidation of the society), and *Yomiuri* "コロナ過剰反応:偏見は社会不安しかうまない" [*Korona kajō hannō: Henken wa shakai fuan shika umanai*] (Overreaction to corona: Prejudice only causes social unrest). The former reminds the reader of the suffering caused by discrimination based on diseases such as leprosy (*Asahi Shimbun*, 2020c). As human rights issues are specifically the justice minister's responsibility, Minister Mori offers support for the victims of corona discrimination and extends this support to victims of domestic violence as an indirect consequence of the pandemic. Nevertheless, Governor Yoshimura is the only leader amongst the four who mentions the word *"shakai"* (society) and urges the community as a whole to create an inclusive society (see Excerpts [7] and [15]). An *Asahi* survey, mentioned earlier (*Asahi Shimbun*, 2020b), placed the governors Yoshimura and Koike as the two most positively evaluated politicians. Governor Koike, with a well-established media profile and the metropolitan government leadership, utilised her sophisticated media self-presentation skills and effective use of strong slogans. Governor Yoshimura, combined with his more direct and personal approach, expressed his community mindedness and seems to have earned positive recognition of his leadership in the pandemic. At the same time, governors are naturally in a position to be closer to the people they represent than are the central government ministers. Further research on the recipients' perceptions of the video messages would help us understand what makes leaders' messages addressing corona discrimination effective.

6. Conclusion

Public announcements play an important role in times of crisis. This chapter has explored how linguistic and semiotic resources are adopted in four political leaders' video messages addressing corona discrimination. The analysis revealed different ways in which the politicians sought cooperation from the public while aligning themselves with their institutional agenda. Their message overall reflected key information and recommendations circulating across public discourse, which ensured credibility. The anti-discrimination messages were also characterised by the use of the war metaphor "fight against the virus," discursively projecting corona discrimination as disruptive to the national unity required in a public health crisis. The leaders' anti-discrimination discourse aimed at countering this highly disruptive discourse of discrimination also implicitly addresses the potential loss of their political power and control. Social stigma and discrimination as a threat to inclusive and compassionate society were not prominently raised despite the fact that disease-based discrimination is a deeply ingrained social issue which the Japanese nation and people need to confront.

Ikuko Nakane is Associate Professor in Japanese at the University of Melbourne. Her research interests include sociolinguistics, discourse analysis, multilingualism, and legal discourse. Her work primarily focuses on negotiation of power and solidarity in institutional discourse. Her articles have appeared in journals such as *Journal of Pragmatics, Semiotica,* and *Multilingua.*

References

Act on Special Measures for Pandemic Influenza and New Infectious Diseases Preparedness and Response 2020. (Japan). Accessed July 10, 2021. https://japan.kantei.go.jp/98_abe/statement/202003/_00001.html.

Asahi Shimbun. 2020a. "Shingata haien, dema ni chuui. 'Tokyo gorin chūshi,' 'chishiritsu 15%.'" [New type of pneumonia, be aware of misinformation: "Tokyo Olympics cancelled," "Mortality rate 15%."] January 1, 2020.

Asahi Shimbun. 2020b. *"Korona taiō, hyōkasuru sējika wa: Ichii wa Yoshimura Osaka fuchiji, nii wa Koike Tokyo tochiji. Asahi Shimbun yoron chōsa"* [Asahi Shinbun survey. Corona response: which politician is highly evaluated? Osaka Governor Yoshimura at the top, Tokyo Governor Koike the 2nd.] December 30, 2020.

Asahi Shimbun. 2020c. *"Korona to sabetsu: Shakai no kōhai o fusegu tame."* [Corona and discrimination: To avoid dilapidation of the society.] April 19, 2020.

Blommaert, Jan. 2005. *Discourse: A Critical Introduction.* Cambridge: Cambridge University Press.

Centre for Human Rights Education and Training 2020. *STOP! Corona Sabetsu: Sabetsu o nakushite tadashii rikai o kyanpēn* [Corona discrimination campaign: Eliminate discrimination and promote a correct understanding]. Accessed 1 July, 2021. http://www.jinken.or.jp/archives/21491.

Chung, Siaw-Fong. 2011. "A corpus-based study of SARS in English news reporting in Malaysia and in the United Kingdom." *International Review of Pragmatics* 3, no. 2: 270–293.

Dada, Sara, Henry Charles Ashworth, Marlene Joannie Bewa, and Roopa Dhatt. 2021. "Words matter: Political and gender analysis of speeches made by heads of government during the COVID-19 pandemic." *BMJ Global Health* 6: e003910.

Dunn, Cynthia Dickel. 2013. "Speaking politely, kindly, and beautifully: Ideologies of politeness in Japanese business etiquette training." *Multilingua: Journal of Cross-Cultural and Interlanguage Communication* 32, no. 2: 225–245.

Eggins, Susanne. 1994. *An Introduction to Systemic Functional Linguistics.* London: Pinter Publishers.

Halliday, Michael. A. K. 1985. *An Introduction to Functional Grammar.* London: Edward Arnold.

Japanese Red Cross Society. 2020. *"Shingata coronauirusu no mittsu no kao o shirō!: Fu no supairaru o tachikiru tameni."* [Get to know the three faces of the novel coronavirus: To break out of a negative spiral.] Accessed July 1, 2021. https://www.jrc.or.jp/saigai/news/200326_006124.html.

Kaneyasu, Michiko. 2019. "The family of Japanese no-wa cleft construction: A register-based analysis." *Lingua* 217: 1–23.

Kimura, Ryoko. 2021. *"Yoshimura Osaka fuchiji no kōhyōka to posutoturūsu jidai."* [Positive evaluation of Osaka Governor Yoshimura and the post-truth era.] *Ronza.* May 12, 2021. https://webronza.asahi.com/culture/articles/2021051100007.html?page=2.

Kress, Gunther R., and Theo van Leeuwen. 2021. *Reading Images: The Grammar of Visual Design.* 3rd ed. Milton: Taylor & Francis Group.

Littlefield, Robert S. 2021. "Controlling the narrative: Mixed messages and presidential credibility." In *Communicating Science in Times of Crisis: COVID-19 Pandemic*, edited by H. Dan O'Hair and Mary John O'Hair, 358–374. Hoboken, NJ: John Wiley & Sons.

Manfredi-Sánchez, Juan-Luis, Adriana Amado-Suárez, and Silvio Waisbord. 2021. "Presidential Twitter in the face of Covid-19: Between populism and pop politics." *Comunicar* 66, no. 29, 83–94.

Ministry of Justice. n.d.. *"Korona sabetsu kaishō ni kansuru hōmushō no torikumi."* [Measures taken by the Ministry of Justice to eliminate corona discrimination.] Accessed July 10, 2021. http://www.moj. go.jp/JINKEN/stop_coronasabetsu.html.

Molnár, Anna, Lili Takács, and Éva Jakusné Harnos. 2020. "Securitization of the COVID-19 pandemic by metaphoric discourse during the State of Emergency in Hungary." *International Journal of Sociology and Social Policy* 40, no. 9/10: 1167–1182.

Nanri, Keizo. 2005. "The conundrum of Japanese editorials: Polarized, diversified and homogeneous." *Japanese Studies* 25, no. 2: 169–185.

O'Hair, H. Dan and Mary John O'Hair. 2021. "Managing science communication in a pandemic." In *Communicating Science in Times of Crisis: COVID-19 Pandemic*, edited by H. Dan O'Hair and Mary John O'Hair, 3–14. Hoboken, NJ: John Wiley & Sons.

Reyes Bernard, Natalie, Abdul Basit, Ernesta Sofija, Hai Phung, Jessica Lee, Shannon Rutherford, Bernadette Sebar, Neil Harris, Dung Phung, and Nicola Wiseman. 2021. "Analysis of crisis communication by the Prime Minister of Australia during the COVID-19 pandemic." *International Journal of Disaster Risk Reduction* 62, no. 1: 102375.

Seargeant, Philip. 2011. "The symbolic meaning of visual English in the social landscape of Japan." In *English in Japan in the Era of Globalization*, edited by Philip Seargeant, 187–204. Basingstoke: Palgrave Macmillan.

Tokyo Metropolitan Government. 2020. "STOP! Korona sabetsu." [Stop! Corona discrimination.] Accessed July 10, 2021. https://www.koho.metro.tokyo.lg.jp/2020/12/09.html.

van Dijk, Teun A. 1993a. "Principles of critical discourse analysis". *Discourse & Society* 4, no. 2: 249–283.

van Dijk, Teun A.1993b. *Elite Discourse and Racism*. Thousand Oaks: SAGE Publications.

van Dijk, Teun A. 1998. "Opinions and ideologies in the press". In *Approaches to Media Discourse*, edited by Allan Bell and Peter Garrett, 21–63. Oxford: Blackwell.

van Dijk, Teun A. 2006. "Discourse and manipulation". *Discourse & Society* 17, no. 3: 359–383.

World Health Organization. n.d. "COVID-19: Addressing social stigma and discrimination." World Health Organization. Accessed August 13, 2021. https://www.who.int/westernpacific/emergencies/ covid-19/information/social-stigma-discrimination.

Yomiuri Shimbun. 2020a. *"Kikokusha taiō seifu kuryo. Bukan daiichibin."* [Government facing difficulties with returnees. First repatriation flight from Wuhan.] January 30, 2020.

Yomiuri Shimbun. 2020b. *"Korona kajō hannō: Henken wa shakai fuan shika umanai."* [Overreaction to corona: Prejudice only causes social unrest.] April 23, 2020.

CHAPTER 6

(Im)politeness of Masked and Non-Masked Faces in the COVID-19 Pandemic: Japan and Australia

Jun Ohashi

Abstract

This chapter examines how perceived social norms and moral concerns for self and others have shaped the discourses and practices of mask wearing during the COVID-19 pandemic. Focusing on how social norms and social identities are formed in online discussion forums in Japan and in Australia, the author thus argues that the topic of (non)mask wearing provides interesting material for the study of interpersonal language and (im)politeness.

Keywords: politeness, impoliteness, masks, social norms, online forum

1. Introduction

The COVID-19 pandemic has been causing unprecedented disruptions all over the world, placing stress on people and society and triggering new behaviours in social life. The wearing of masks, which also symbolises and visualises the prolonged COVID-19 pandemic around the globe, is one such behaviour. Historical, sociocultural, and political factors seem to have an impact on the habit of mask wearing, which has spread quickly in some countries, not so quickly in others.

The decision-making process of wearing or not wearing a mask involves social actors' consideration of "doing the right thing" in terms of perceived social norms, peer pressure, moral obligations, sense of security, concern for others, and public self-image. Therefore, the topic of (non-)mask wearing provides rich material for the study of interpersonal pragmatics and (im)politeness, which investigates interpersonal mutual evaluation and face work during a disruptive public-health crisis.

Online discussion forums illuminate laypersons' attitudes and emotions about (non-)mask wearing. These places offer a platform where individuals can express their attitudes and emotions regarding the topics posted. Few studies to date, however, have explored meaning making in discussion forums representing lay perspectives on mask wearing. To examine the question of how social actors position themselves in relation to (non-)mask wearing, Ohashi (2021) analyses the discourse of (non-)mask wearing in an online discussion forum. The analysis demonstrated how participants evaluate (non-)mask wearing behaviours and form social identities and social norms through their comment making practices.

This chapter furthers that work by including a cross-cultural perspective, comparing popular social media platforms in Australia and Japan. In Australia, mask mandates varied from state to state. In Melbourne, the first region to mandate mask wearing, masks were made compulsory from July 23, 2020 and hard-line measures, including a 112-day lockdown, were taken to prevent a second wave of infections. Since then, wearing masks quickly became the norm. In Japan, on the other hand, masks have never been compulsory; despite this, most people wear them in public. Also, unlike Australia, Japan had a lenient policy to contain this highly contagious disease (i.e., minimal testing, voluntary lockdowns, no domestic travel bans, etc.).

This study aims to elucidate how social actors engage with each other on the topic of mask wearing on social media platforms, how they position themselves and others, and how they form social identities in the "here and now" from a cross-cultural perspective. Findings are expected to benefit the study of interpersonal pragmatics where theorising (im)politeness and face work (public self-image management) are of major concern.

Following some background information on the COVID-19 pandemic, especially in relation to the habit of mask wearing in Australia and Japan, I will present earlier research on masks in the pandemic to identify knowledge gaps and formulate research questions, which will be followed by a description of the theoretical framework, data, and the method of analysis.

2. Background

According to the COVID-19 Behaviour Tracker produced by the Institute of Global Health Innovation, Imperial College London with polling company YouGov, Japan and Australia exhibit very different pictures in terms of mask-wearing habits. During the period June 22 to June 28, 2020, in response to the statement "I have worn a face mask outside my home," of 1,000 Japanese respondents 77% answered "always," and 9% "frequently," whereas their Australian counterparts were 10% and 9% respectively. An even starker difference is shown amongst those who responded "not at all," with 64% of Australians giving this response compared to a mere 3% of Japanese. Put simply, mask wearing was the norm in Japan but not in Australia at that time. This quickly shifted in Melbourne, however, when the wearing of masks became compulsory on July 23, 2020, with the threat of an AU$200 fine for non-compliance. This financial threat may have been one of the causes leading to increased mask wearing in Melbourne. Japan on the other hand puzzled major foreign media including the BBC and The Guardian for its high degree of mask-wearing compliance with minimal intervention from the government.[1] In Japan, masks have never been compulsory, but a majority of people still wear them (Tsukimoro, 2021).

As early as March 26, 2020, the media depicted Japan's management of the virus as successful given their low infection rates and fatalities. The *New York Times* published an article describing Japan as having "only 1,300 cases and 45 deaths reported, with one of the slowest-progressing death rates in the world despite its aging population" and describing Japan as being in a state of "business as usual" (Rich and Ueno, 2020). At the time, the BBC depicted Japan's low virus death rate as mysterious, and suspected it was related to the fact that "the government can count on the public to comply" and that "Japan asked people to take care, stay away from crowded places, wear masks and wash their hands—and by and large, that is exactly what most people have done" (Wingfield-Hayes, 2020).

Foreign media depictions of Japan quickly became a catalyst for rather naive cross-cultural analyses with nationalistic intent. Predictably, then Prime Minister Shinzo Abe quickly seized the moment to boast of Japan's success, as did Finance Minister Taro Aso. On June 4, 2020 to praise the people of Japan, Aso commented that the lower fatality rate in comparison to other advanced economies was due to Japan's higher "level of cultural standards" (民度のレベルが違う) (The Japan Times, 2020).

Interestingly The Guardian reported on October 27, 2020 that Japan was ranked lowest in government approval ratings (21%) even though the coronavirus death rate was one of the lowest, stating "only 21% of Japanese respondents said they felt their government had handled the crisis very or fairly well" (Henley and Barr, 2020). The low approval rating suggests that Abe's and Aso's statements praising the people would have been interpreted as empty political statements to mask the government's inaction.

3. Images of Masks in the COVID-19 Pandemic

What images, then, do people have in regard to the wearing of face masks? Ji (2020) analysed nine government-sponsored anti-epidemic videos released in China to examine how they build face-mask-related narratives. Ji's analysis reveals that:

> "face mask in use" links people's "smaller love" for their family to a "bigger love" for Chinese people in general; transforms an individual to member of a large group of commoner-turned-protectors; or marks the military's loyalty and obedience to the Party-State, which makes possible the "Chinese speed" in saving lives. (p. 6)

Ji (2020) also touches upon the legacy of Confucianism, which still influences the Chinese psyche in relation to mask-wearing compliance:

> Confucianism did not simply induce submission to authorities. It is the synergy between Confucianism's family-state complex and China's cultural inclination to moralize and emotionalize public issues that provides the narrative with legitimacy and persuasiveness. (p. 6)

Nakayachi et al. (2020) conducted a survey between March 26 and March 31, 2020 involving 1,000 (F:515, M:485) participants across all age groups above 20 years of age to examine why people adopted mask wearing. The survey results concluded that Japanese participants' mask-wearing behaviours are motivated by conformity to social norm, rather than by wanting to reduce their risk of being infected or spreading the virus to others. In other words, Japanese masked faces represent more their conformity induced by peer pressure. The results may imply the legacy of Confucianism in Japan, not in terms of "submission to authorities" (Ji, 2020, p. 6), but rather the values of group harmony (Dollinger, 1988) and conformity to social norms.[2]

Sakakibara and Ozono (2020), on the other hand, draw a different conclusion in a similar study conducted between April 28 and May 5, 2020, involving 3,892 (F:1771, M:2121, range 18–86 years) participants. They conclude that people tend to wear masks to prevent infection of themselves and others, rather than conformity to others' mask-wearing behaviours. Sakakibara and Ozono (2021) critically assess the inconsistent results by conducting another survey (F:559, M:721, Others:7) incorporating some new survey questions. They argue that both the conformity to the social norm and autonomous decision-making to reduce the risk of being infected and giving the virus to others are significant to making sense of mask-wearing behaviours in Japan. Sakakibara and Ozono (2021) speculate that the inconsistent results from the two studies are due to the timing of the surveys. Then Prime Minister Abe declared a state of emergency in seven prefectures (Tokyo, Kanagawa, Saitama, Chiba, Osaka, Hyogo, and Fukuoka) on April 7, 2020, and expanded the scope to the entire nation on April 16.[3] Nakayachi et al. (2020) conducted the survey before the state of emergency was declared by the Japanese government, whereas the survey by Sakakibara and Ozono (2020) was conducted after the declaration. Sakakibara and Ozono (2021) explain that the general public's sense of threat to the spread of the virus increased after the declaration of the state of emergency, and thus the survey conducted by Sakakibara and Ozono (2020) after the declaration indicates a stronger tendency towards an autonomous decision to wear masks. It is still unclear whether people wear masks to prevent infection of themselves and/ or others or simply to conform to others' mask-wearing behaviours; however, as Sakakibara and Ozono (2021) point out, the social and political context of the time influences the public's decisions.

Mask wearing has been employed by many countries as a measure to combat COVID-19. The prevailing attitudes of the general public towards mask wearing— in other words, social norms—identify what is deviant (Inglis and Almila, 2020). There is research being carried out on the development of databases and systems to identify deviants, people who are not wearing masks correctly (Batagelj et al., 2021; Cabani et al., 2021). However, there are few studies on what the general public thinks and feels about wearing or not wearing masks in the COVID-19 pandemic through their participation in online discussion forums, even though the general public express their sentiment significantly more on online forums than other social media such as Instagram or Facebook (Chang et al. 2020). Ohashi (2021) is an exception, focusing on a discussion thread in an online social community, sharing participants' opinions and experiences of their wearing/not wearing masks immediately after mask wearing was made mandatory by the state government of Victoria in Australia. Ohashi observes that participants contribute to the creation of ever-changing social norms, and that even simple evaluative language plays an important role in creating social norms and group-oriented social identities.

Understanding social and psychological aspects of social actors' reflections regarding (non-)mask wearing is significant for policy makers who wish to promote mask-wearing compliance. This chapter builds on Ohashi's (2021) study by asking the following questions from a cross-cultural perspective:

- How do discussion forum participants in Japan and Australia evaluate (non-) mask-wearing behaviours?
- How do they claim their position, "pro-mask" or "anti-mask"?
- Are there any culturally specific or similar phenomena shared between the target discussion threads, one dealing with (non-)mask-wearing behaviours in Japan and the other in Australia?

4. Theoretical Framework

In order to explore these questions, I draw on the following theoretical assumptions.

4.1 Social Norms

Social norms influence people's behaviours and perceptions, and it is important to take account of the notion of social norms to make sense of how participants talk about masks in social media. Drawing on Elster (1989), social norms are understood here as "emotional and behavioural propensities of individuals" (p. 102). Thus, these social norms are emergent and fluid. They reside not only in social but also psychological domains of human activities, in other words they are "shared by other people and partly sustained by their approval and disapproval" (ibid., pp. 99–100) and "by the feelings of embarrassment, anxiety, guilt and shame that a person suffers at the prospect of violating them" (ibid., p. 100). Both domains influence human behaviours: "information about what others think one should do (injunctive norms) and what they actually do (descriptive norms) has been shown to crucially influence individuals' decisions to think and/or behave in particular ways" (Steentjes et al., 2017, p. 117). Perceived social norms give social actors legitimacy to behave and speak certain ways in a given time and space.

4.2 Attitude and Stance

In Elster's (1989) model of social norms, approval or disapproval by social actors is considered to influence one's perception of social norms. Social actors' (dis)approval is manifested linguistically. I draw on Martin's (2004) definition of "attitude," which is often manifested adjectivally and conveys emotions ("affect"), evaluations ("judgement") or preference ("appreciation"). Attitude functions relationally in interpersonal communication, and its linguistic manifestation positions a social actor in relation to addressees, principles, or social norms. A more dynamic understanding of attitude in interaction is "stance":

> Stance is a public act by a social actor, achieved dialogically through overt communicative means, of simultaneously evaluating objects, positioning subjects (self and others), and aligning with other subjects, with respect to any salient dimension of the sociocultural field. (Du Bois, 2007, p. 163)

Du Bois (2007) uses the concept of the stance triangle to explicate the mechanism of stance taking. From the first-person point of view, he describes the essence of it: "I evaluate something, and thereby position myself, and thereby align with you" (p. 163). Expressing one's opinion or evaluation about a topic in a discussion forum, for instance, is stance taking because it indicates one's position and clarifies one's relation to others. Myers (2010) goes a little further to claim that stance taking "involves using that opinion to align or disalign with someone else" (p. 264).

4.3 (Im)politeness

The notion of (im)politeness as an evaluative mechanism is one of the key foci of the study of interpersonal pragmatics (Kádár and Haugh, 2013; Watts, 2003). (Im)politeness is used as a notional continuum scale to capture both positive and negative evaluations made by participants. Therefore, the terms "impoliteness" and "politeness" will not be used as a priori labels unless participants use either of them to evaluate themselves or their interlocutors. Goffman's (1967, p. 5) notion of face—"the positive social value a person effectively claims for himself [*sic*] by the line others assume he has taken during a particular contact"—is often assumed by post-Brown and Levinsonian scholars of (im)politeness research. This study also employs Goffman's understanding of face and assumes that participants care for their own positive public self-image, and that they exchange comments "in particular ways by which they achieve a good and pleasant self-evaluation and public self-image" (Ohashi, 2008, p. 2171). It is also assumed that the "particular ways" reflect emergent and dynamic (micro-)cultural social norms (Elster, 1989).

This line of thinking is based on the assumption that the construal of "self" is interdependent. It is conceptualised as "a constellation of thoughts, feelings, and actions concerning one's relationship to others, and self as distinct from others" (Singelis, 1994, p. 581), and herein I assume the view of interdependent construal of self which Markus and Kitayama (1991) define as inclination:

> seeing oneself as part of an encompassing **social relationship** and recognizing that one's behaviour is determined, contingent on, and, to a large extent organized by what the actor perceives to be the thoughts, feelings, and actions of others in the **relationship**. (Markus and Kitayama 1991, p. 227; emphasis added)

I argue that social identities and social norms are closely related in the sense that the symbolic meaning of mask wearing involves people's understanding of, and enacting of, social norms with which they position and categorise themselves and others.

According to social identity theory (Turner et al., 1987; Tajfel and Turner, 1986), people accentuate intergroup differences—in other words, they amplify the positive attributes of their perceived in-group members in contrast to those who are perceived as out-group members in order for the in-group members to attain positive social identity.

5. Data and Analyses

Data for the study are two major social media discussion forums: one is populated by users who share interest in issues regarding Melbourne and Australia in general, the other is one of the biggest Japanese online discussion forums. For convenience and clarity, I will refer to the former as A-forum and the latter as J-forum. Ohashi (2021) conducted a preliminary investigation of A-Forum, on which this chapter will build to draw a comparison with J-forum. The number of comments amounts to 756 in A-forum and 537 in J-forum; Table 1 below summarises key information about the targeted discussion forums.

Table 1: Discussion Forums to be Investigated

	A-forum	J-forum
Number of posts	756	537
Duration of the activity	July 25, 2020–July 27, 2020	Nov 2, 2020–June 15, 2021
Local situations related to the COVID-19 pandemic	Number of new cases: 437 on July 25 in Australia. Three days after the Victoria State Government in Australia announced a mask-wearing mandate for the first time in metropolitan Melbourne. The number of new cases increased until it hit a record high of 715 cases on August 5, 2020. The number quickly decreased, and October 16 marked no new cases.	Number of new cases: 488 on November 2 in Japan. Gradually the number increased until it hit a record high on January 8, 2021, marking 7,863 new cases a day in Japan. The number decreased quickly until March 6 (412 new cases) and increased again to hit another high (7,521) on May 12, 2021.
Content of the initial post	"I'm kinda proud of Melbourne right now." The statement expressed the poster's joy of witnessing people in Melbourne comply with the mask-wearing mandate quickly.	"最近、マスクしていない奴が多すぎると思わね？" [*saikin masuku shitenai **yatsu** ga oosugiru to omowane?*] (Don't you think there are too many **people** [derog.] who don't wear masks these days?) The poster raised his/her concerns with people not wearing masks.

In order to see participants' attitudes towards mask wearing in each forum, the linguistic manifestation of their attitudes is investigated in relation to the research questions, "How do discussion forum participants in Japan and Australia evaluate (non-)mask-wearing behaviours?" and "How do they claim their position, 'pro-mask' or 'anti-mask?"

Du Bois's (2007) stance triangle is employed to make sense of the data. In the context of discussion forums, the stance triangle is modified as – the poster, the stancetaker, evaluates pro- or anti-maskers and/or their behaviours and thereby positions him/herself, and thereby aligns/disaligns with target audience (pro- or anti-maskers) in the discussion forum in question.

In the sections to follow, frequently occurring lexical items which manifest posters' attitudes including evaluative predicates and address terms towards intended audience (pro- or anti-maskers) and towards (non-)mask-wearing behaviours are identified, and NVivo is used to perform quantitative and qualitative analysis.

5.1 A-forum

A person posted a comment with the title: "I'm kinda proud of Melbourne right now," and s/he describes many people wearing masks three days after face coverings were mandated (an AU$200 fine was applied to noncompliance in metropolitan Melbourne).

Frequently occurring lexical items attributable to "attitude" or "stance" were identified first, and Table 2 below illustrates adjectives and adjectival nouns which allow participants to evaluate and take a stance on (non-)masking-related behaviours, alongside some examples. Positive and negative evaluative lexical items are both present, but there is no guarantee that their form and lexical meaning will match the addresser's intent or addressee's interpretation, and so it is necessary to qualitatively analyse the data. All listed lexical items appeared more than ten times except for "stupid" (six times), but it is included for its semantic proximity to "idiot." Since "good" and "great" and also "proud" and "happy" are functionally similar to each other, they are analysed together.

Table 2: Frequently Occurring Evaluative Predicates and Address Terms in A-forum

Adjectives/ adjectival nouns	Count	Example
Good	39	"**Good** work, Melbourne!"
Great	16	"Victoria is doing **great**"
Proud	15	"I'm so **proud** of everyone!
Happy	12	"(I) was **happy** to see really good compliance overall"
Bad	19	"a really **bad** idea"
Idiot	11	"I've only seen the occasional **idiot** who puts their own comfort above the wellbeing of the community"
Stupid	6	"Are they **stupid** and actually think that it is how a mask works"

5.1.1 Good (39) and Great (16)

The most frequent term is "good" as in "**Good** work, Melbourne!" "**Good** to see," "Masks are pretty **good** yeah," "**good** going Melbs" to commend fellow Melburnians for wearing masks. Such uses of "good" directly and positively evaluate mask-wearing behaviours, and clearly indicate the posters' pro-mask position. In terms of Du

Bois's (2007) notion of the stance triangle, the majority of the posters are pro-maskers and they evaluate pro-maskers and their behaviours positively, thereby positioning themselves as pro-maskers, and thereby aligning with other pro-maskers. However, some phrases such as "**good** point" and another use of "**good** work" in a different context are not evaluating mask-wearing behaviours but are acknowledging and praising comments and information posted by other contributors. Such uses of "good" are relationally effective, but do not necessarily indicate a pro-mask position. "Good" appeared in the phrase "more harm than **good**" twice by different posters who claimed that touching a mask or wearing a mask inappropriately is problematic, but still thought wearing one was better than not. "Good" does not necessarily evaluate mask-wearing behaviours but it is at least relationally significant. "Great" is used similarly to "good" but was usually tied to positive evaluation of mask-wearing behaviours, for example, "Victoria is doing **great**," "**great** we wear masks," "**great** to see," and "it's been **great**," all of which refer to mask wearing.

5.1.2 Proud (15) and Happy (12)

"Proud" and "happy" are affective predicates which position the stancetakers affectively (Du Bois, 2007, p. 143) expressing their positive evaluation of fellow Melburnians' compliance to mask wearing. Examples of the use of "proud" include, "such a **proud** day for me," "I am so **proud** of everyone!" "we can feel **proud** of our city again," and "so **proud** of my hometown." Some uses of "proud" appear to be closely related to a poster's sense of community, as in "I'm so **proud** of everyone! I feel like it's bringing us all closer together in some way... helping us connect as a community." Such inclusive vocabulary as "us," "closer together," "connect" and "community" also co-occurred. Another participant echoed this comment in writing "this is why Melbourne is going to kill this sucker quickly and efficiently. So **proud** of my hometown." Through comments like these a pro-mask stance is consolidated. There are two posts which question those who are "proud" of Melburnians' compliance to mask wearing. They do not challenge nor criticise mask-wearing compliance itself, but they are not proud of it either because, as one argues, "it took a mandatory mask order to get people to wear masks" and the other "legal obligation was the only way to motivate people," both reflecting on their fellow Melburnians' lack of voluntary mask wearing at earlier stages of the pandemic.

Similar to the use of "proud," "happy" is also used to express participants' positive attitudes towards mask-wearing compliance. Some examples include "**happy** to see the masked faces when I'm out walking," "[100% compliance] makes me **happy**," "**happy** to be seeing masks around." "Not **happy**" is used to express participants' critical stance on a chosen issue. A participant criticises those who visit the surf coast from Melbourne during the lockdown by stating, "I'm not very happy." Another participant states that "a lot of people aren't **happy** about it" to align with those who are critical about the AU$200 fine.

5.1.3 Bad (19)

"Bad" expresses participants' negative attitude towards a chosen topic. It was used on a variety of topics, not only in relation to (non-)mask-wearing behaviours: "a really **bad** idea," referring to someone not wearing a mask, but also the consequences of the health response to the COVID-19 pandemic, including the increasing number of new cases in the US, leadership in the US, and negative economic impact. The data show that "bad" was used in wide ranging subtopics.

5.1.4 Idiot (11) and Stupid (6)

"Idiot" and "stupid" were mainly used to refer to anti-maskers or non-mask-wearing behaviours in this discussion forum. They are derogatory labels or terms of address with which addressers position themselves by othering or identifying out-group members, while claiming a pro-mask stance. "Idiot" was mainly used in this thread to refer to those who do not conform to the mask-wearing mandate. For instance, one participant has "seen the occasional **idiot** who puts their own comfort above the wellbeing of the community." A supermarket employee reported that "we've only had one **idiot** customer come in without a mask." A participant who totally forgot about wearing a mask at a nearby pizza takeaway shop "feel[s] like a complete **idiot**." There is one instance of the use referring to those who wear masks, "all these **idiots** wearing masks thinking they deserve a fucken Medal & shaming others." Though the use of "idiot" is closely related to non-masked people and their behaviours, the use of "stupid" is more general, enough to cover US government policies on the COVID-19 pandemic. There are three counts of "stupid" and two counts of "moron" referring to those who do not fully comply with the mask mandate. Such derogatory terms are predominantly used in the thread to disapprove of those who do not comply with the mask-wearing mandate, and to claim a pro-mask identity. The more negative evaluations are attached to people not wearing masks, the more such negative views are consolidated as social norms within this community.

While there is no way of confirming exactly what motivated more Melburnians to wear masks during this time, sensitivity to emerging social norms may have been one of the significant influencing factors. Combining positive and negative terms such as good, great, happy, proud, bad, idiot, and stupid, social actors express their attitudes to the issues on social media, and position themselves (or take a stance) and form a social identity. Social norms are formed and contested as users continue to post their views and reactions to them.

5.2 J-forum

A person initiated a thread with the title: "マスクしない奴に対する規制についてどう思う？" [*Masuku shinai yatsu ni tai suru kisei ni tsuite dou omou?*] (What do you think about restrictions on people who don't wear masks?) and continued as follows.

> 1. 最近、マスクしていない奴が多すぎると思わね？
>
> ヨーロッパの様になる前に規制は必要だと思うんだけどさ。
>
> みんなはどう思う？
>
> [*Saikin, masuku shitenai yatsu ga ōsugiru to omowane?*
>
> *Yōroppa no yōni naru mae ni kisei wa hitsuyōda to omoundakedo sa.*
>
> *Minna wa dō omou?*]
>
> (Too many people are not wearing masks these days, don't you think?
>
> I think we need to regulate this before we become like Europe.
>
> What do you guys think?)

In J-forum, address terms and second-person pronouns dominated as shown in Table 3 below. This may be attributable to the fact that address terms and personal pronouns are significant relation-acknowledging devices in the Japanese language (Ishiyama, 2019).

Table 3: Frequently Occurring Evaluative Predicates and Address Terms in J-forum

Adjectives/ adjectival nouns	Count	Examples
奴 (71) やつ (13) ヤツ (1) *Yatsu* (person [derog.]: a bloke, dude, bastard, jerk)	85	"マスクつける奴は俺が許さない" [*Masuku tsukeru yatsu wa ore ga yurusanai*] (I won't forgive any **bastards** who wear a mask)
お前 *Omae* (you [derog.])	47	"お前みたいな病気を舐めてる奴の意見を聞くのが馬鹿らしいよ" [***Omae** mitaina byōki wo nameteru yatsu no iken wo kikuno ga baka rashī yo*] (It's ridiculous to listen to people like **you [derog.]** who take the disease so lightly)
バカ (22) 馬鹿 (16) *Baka* (idiot/ stupid)	38	"ほんとバカだなマスク勢って" [*Honto **baka** dana masuku zeitte*] (The mask people are really **stupid**)

Adjectives/ adjectival nouns	Count	Examples
アホ (17) あほ (2) *Aho* (idiot/ stupid)	19	"問題になってるのは故意にマスクをしないアホ" [*Mondai ni natteruno wa koini masuku wo shinai **aho***] (It's the **idiots** who deliberately don't wear masks that are the problem).
迷惑 *Meiwaku* (annoyance)	18	"マスクは他人に迷惑をかけないためにするんだよ" [*Masuku wa tanin ni **meiwaku** wo kakenai tameni surunda yo*] (Masks are for not **bothering** others)
悪い *Warui* (bad)	15	"マスクしない奴が圧倒的に悪い" [*Masuku shinai **yatsu** ga attōtekini **warui***] (**Bastards** who don't wear masks are by far the **worst**)

Frequently occurring linguistic items which indicate the poster's position regarding (non-)mask wearing in the J-forum, where address terms occupied the top two positions, illuminate a very different picture to the A-forum. Japanese personal pronouns have been characterised as very different to those of English—in fact, Suzuki (1978) argues that using the term "personal pronouns" as a grammatical category in Japanese is misleading, as it does not capture the function of the phenomenon in Japanese, and that they should be placed, along with "kinship terms, position terms, etc., into the categories of all words used by the speaker with reference to himself [*sic*] and to the addressee" (Suzuki, 1978, p. 93).

There are multiple ways to address oneself in Japanese, including *watakushi, watashi, atashi, boku, ore, jibun,* and so forth, depending on the formality of a given occasion, the interlocutor, social role assigned in a given context and so on. Similarly, there are a variety of second-person pronouns such as *anata, anta, kimi, kisama, omae, otaku, temē,* and so on (See Ishiyama [2019] for historical accounts of personal pronouns as relation-acknowledging devices). Such varieties of first and second-person pronouns and an elaborate honourification system in Japanese suggest that positioning self, the addressee, and referents is of great importance. Therefore, personal pronouns and address terms are of great significance in stance taking (Du Bois, 2007). Given that first-person pronouns are highly elliptical in Japanese, second/third pronouns and addressee terms are significant in indicating the position of the addresser in relation to the addressee and others in the interaction.

5.2.1 Yatsu (85)

Yatsu appears in three different forms, 奴, (in *kanji*, logographic Chinese character), やつ (in *hiragana* syllabaries), and ヤツ (in *katakana* syllabaries). Their counts are 71, 13 and 1 respectively. 奴 is a derogatory term which originally meant a servant, and it is translated variously depending on context. Common English counterparts include, "bloke," "dude," "bastard," or "jerk." In this thread, *yatsu* is predominantly used to refer to those who do not wear a mask, as in *masuku shinai/shitenai yatsu* (a bastard who does not wear a mask), which occurred 14 times. *Masuku shiteru/tsukeru yatsu* (a bastard who wears a mask) occurred twice including the example in Table 3.

5.2.2 Omae (47)

Omae appears 47 times. According to スーパー大辞林 [*Super Daijirin*] (2020), *omae* was written as 御前, and used as a second-person pronoun referring to the presence of a deity, a Buddha, or a nobleman with respect in ancient times. The word was eventually used as a respectful way of addressing a noble person, without directly referring to him or her. It also came to be used as a second-person pronoun. In the mid-Edo period, the aspect of respect implicit in the term was lost to a great extent, and it continued to be lost after that, until it came to be used not only for peers but also for subordinates, as it is today.[4] It can be used online as a condescending term of address.

In this thread, *omae* was used by both pro- and anti-mask participants when they attack their opponents, indicating impoliteness. The following examples illustrate how お前 [*omae*] and お前ら [*omaera* pl.] are used in context.

> 2. それでも俺はノーマスクを貫き、お前らみたいなマスク狂と戦って行くぜw
>
> [*Soredemo ore wa nōmasuku wo tsuranuki, omaera mitai na masukukyō to tatakatte ikuze*]
>
> (But I'm still going to wear no mask and fight against mask crazies like **you (derog.)** ha)

The poster declared that s/he will fight against the opponent, pro-mask people who are described as マスク狂 [*masuku kyō*] (mask crazies).

> 3. 感染症をうつす確率を高めると判ってて他人の直近でノーマスクでいるのは人によっては生命を脅かす暴力なんだからそれを権利だと主張すればお前の論理は破綻する
>
> [*Kansenshō wo utsusu kakuritsu wo takameruto wakattete tanin no chokkin de nōmasuku de iruno wa hito ni yotte wa seimei wo obiyakasu bōryoku nandakara sore wo kenri dato shuchōsureba omae no riron wa hatan suru*]
>
> (Wearing no mask in the vicinity of others when you know it increases the chance of transmitting infection is life-threatening violence to some people, so if you claim it as a right, **your (derog.)** logic falls apart)

As use of *omae* signals the poster's attitude of patronising superiority, it gives rise to impoliteness. There are 20 pro-mask posts and 16 anti-mask posts containing one or more *omae*.

5.2.3 Baka (38)

Baka appears 22 times as バカ in *katakana*, 16 times as馬鹿 in kanji. *Baka* is an adjectival noun, and there are many theories about its origin. According to 日本大百科全書 [*Nihon Dai Hyakka Zensho*] 18 (Shougakukan, 1994), the word is said to be a corruption of the Sanskrit words *moha* (慕何, foolishness) and *mahalaka* (摩訶羅, ignorance), but it is also said to be a corruption of the word *bakka* (破家, foolish to the point of destroying the family property). In any case *baka* equates to "idiot" in English.

> 4. 他人にマスク強要するバカはネット上にしかいないしね
>
> [*Tanin ni masuku kyōyō suru **baka** wa netto jō ni shika inaishi ne*
>
> (**Idiots** who force others to wear masks only exist on the Internet)
>
> 5. 他人のノーマスクが気になって仕方がないバカはよっぽどマスクしたくないんだなw
>
> [*Tanin no nōmasuku ga kini natte shikataganai **baka** wa yoppodo masuku shitaku nainda na*]
>
> (The **idiots** who are so bothered by other people's no-masking really don't want to wear masks ha)
>
> 6. 電車内でマスクつけずに、何かに怒り狂って一人でヤイヤイ言ってるバカがいたけど大迷惑。
>
> [*Denshanai de masuku tsukezuni nanika ikarikurutte hitoride yaiyai itteru **baka** ga itakedo daimeiwaku*]
>
> (There was an **idiot** on the train who didn't wear a mask and was yapping all by himself because he was angry about something, and it was a big nuisance)
>
> 7. 年末年始に大勢でマスク外して飲み食いした馬鹿が多いだけだろ
>
> [*Nenmatsu nenshi ni ōzeide masuku hazushite nomikuishita **baka** ga ōi dake darō*]
>
> (It's just a lot of **idiots** eating and drinking with their masks off in large numbers over the New Year holidays)

Both pro- and anti-maskers use *baka* equally to attack their opponents.

5.2.4 Aho (19)

Aho appeared predominantly in katakana (アホ). According to the online 語源由来辞典 [*Gogen Yurai Jiten*], one of the most popular theories for the word is that Zen monks introduced *aho*, a word meaning "silly" in the Jiangnan region of China, and that the Japanese reading of the word became *ahau*, which in turn became *aho*. The meaning of *aho* and *baka* are considered to be very similar; *aho* means a foolish person or a foolish behaviour. In the Kansai area, however, it is considered less offensive than *baka*. Both pro-and anti-maskers use *aho* to attack the opposition.

In reacting to a post which raises concerns about those who cannot wear masks due to their medical conditions, the following post targets those who deliberately do not wear masks by labelling them アホ [*aho*].

> 8. 問題になってるのは故意にマスクをしないアホであって病気や障害でマスクを着けられない人達じゃないから
>
> [*Mondai ni natteruno wa koini masuku wo shinai **aho** deatte byōki ya shōgai de masuku wo tsukerarenai hitotachi janai kara*]
>
> (It's the **idiots** who deliberately don't wear masks that are the problem, not the people who can't wear them because of illness or disability)

In response to the following post, which demands an answer to the question "Why is the number of infected people increasing when everyone is wearing masks?"

> 9. みんなマスクしてるね〜じゃあなんで増えてるの???
>
> [*Minna masuku shiterune ~ jā nande fueteruno???*]
>
> (Everyone's wearing masks—so why is there an increase???)

A participant responded as follows:

> 10. お前みたいなアホがいるからだって気付けwwwwwwwwwww [*Omae mitaina **aho** ga iru-kara date kizuke*]
>
> (Realise it's because of **idiots** like **you (derog.)**! ha ha ha ha ha ha ha ha ha)

In this interaction the participant questioning the increase in COVID-19 cases was quickly labelled a non-mask idiot. Such derogatory address terms are used in this instance to other the opponent and take a pro-mask stance. The seemingly inno-cent question, which does not clearly position the poster as anti-mask is quickly retaliated with *omae* and *aho*. Derogatory address terms contribute to a binary divide and diminish a space for building common ground or having meaningful information exchanges.

5.2.5 Meiwaku (18)

According to スーパー大辞林 [*Super Daijirin*] (2020), 迷惑 [*meiwaku*] means being offended or annoyed by the behaviour of others. It originally meant being lost, confused, or unsure of what to do, but is now commonly used to raise awareness of undesirable behaviour in public places. The first example illustrates a poster's frustration towards the Japanese government's lenient approach to dealing with the pandemic. The poster stated マジ迷惑 (seriously annoying) because restaurants and bars are potentially helping spread the virus, but they were never closed.

11. 飲食店は強制閉鎖令出すべきマジ迷惑

[*Inshokuten wa kyōsei heisarei dasubeki maji **meiwaku***]

(There should be a mandatory closure order for restaurants. Seriously **annoying**)

The next two examples of the use of *meiwaku* identify undesirable behaviour of non-mask wearing in public space.

12. マスクは他人に迷惑をかけないためにするんだよ。この国には、「人に迷惑をかける自由」はない

[*Masuku wa tanin ni **meiwaku** wo kakenai tameni surunda yo. Konokuni ni wa "hito ni **meiwaku** wo kakeru jiyū" wa nai*]

(We wear masks so that we don't **bother** others. There is no "freedom to **bother** others" in this country)

13. そういう身勝手な奴が二割もいるから 他の八割が迷惑するんだよ

[*Sōyū migattena yatsu ga niwarimo irukara hokano hachiwari ga **meiwaku** surunda yo*]

(It's the 20% who are selfish that **annoy** the other 80%)

5.2.6 Warui (15)

悪い [*warui*] is an adjective meaning "bad." It is used to evaluate something negatively, and in this thread the term is predominantly used by pro-mask participants to argue against non-mask-wearing behaviour. Another key word, 迷惑 [*meiwaku*], defined above, is used to frame non-mask wearing as public misbehaviour.

14. マスクをしていない方が悪い!

[*Masuku wo shiteinai hō ga **warui!***]

(Not wearing a mask is **worse**!)

15. 今のご時世マスクしない奴が圧倒的に悪い他人からしたら迷惑極まりない

[*Ima no gojisei masuku shinai **yatsu** ga attōtekini **warui** tanin karashitara **meiwaku** kiwamarinai*]

(People who don't wear masks are by far the **worst** in the current climate. They are a complete **nuisance** to others)

Warui is also used in the phrase 気持ち悪い [*kimochi warui*] meaning "disgusting." It occurs 5 times, examples include:

16. 俺は寄ってかないから寧ろノーマスクの方が距離感近くて気持ち悪いわ

[*Ore wa yottekanai kara mushiro nōmasuku no hō ga kyorikan chikakute kimochi **warui** wa*]

(I don't come close to them, but no-maskers come close to me and it's **disgusting**)

17. マスクして無い奴らって気持ち悪い顔さしてる

[*Masuku shite nai **yatsura** tte kimochi **warui** kaosa shiteru*]

(Those **bastards** who don't wear masks have **disgusting** faces)

The uses of *warui* contribute to the negative assessment of various behaviours and attributes of anti-maskers in this thread.

6. Discussion

The study in this chapter illustrates the participants' reactions to (non-) mask-wearing behaviour in two discussion forums in a different time and space. Findings will be discussed in relation to the first two research questions, "How do discussion forum participants in Japan and Australia evaluate (non-)mask-wearing behaviours?" and "How do they claim their position, 'pro-mask' or 'anti-mask'?"

In the A-forum, the initial post, "I'm kinda proud of Melbourne right now" may have set the tone and attracted like-minded people. It is a reflection of a specific context in Melbourne where the first mask-wearing mandate was announced by the state government and Melburnians quickly adopted the new habit. They joined the thread and quickly formed a social norm which would legitimate the pro-mask comments, using adjectives such as "good," 'great', 'proud' and 'happy' to positively evaluate the mask-wearing behaviour they observed. They publicly displayed their attitude and positions with such linguistic devices to form pro-mask identity. Pro-maskers negatively evaluated anti-mask behaviours, using "bad," "idiot" and "stupid" to enhance their pro-mask social identity.

In the J-forum, the initial poster raised his/her concerns about growing numbers of non-masked people in public places. Wearing a mask is recommended by the Japanese government but has never been mandatory. Unlike Australia, however, the wearing of masks was not an entirely new practice in Japan, and people were compliant from the early stages of the pandemic. Derogatory address terms were used to other the opponent, and contribute to creating the confrontational and polarised tone of the thread. These terms instantly and clearly revealed participants' attitudes and positions towards (non-)mask wearing, and thus the actual stating of opinions was not essential to take a stance in this thread. The use of *meiwaku* (annoyance and nuisance) to identify unacceptable behaviours in public places was unique to the J-forum. It was not simply expressing annoyance with regard to a targeted behaviour, but was demanding conformity to the desired social norms of the addresser.

Regarding the third research question, "Are there any culturally specific or similar phenomena between the two online discussion forums?" the forums presented more differences than similarities. The A-forum contained frequently occurring positive evaluative lexical items, but the J-forum did not. In the A-forum, there were no confrontational posts calling users derogatory address terms, targeting a specific audience. However, derogatory address terms tended to be used by pro-maskers to consolidate their pro-mask social identity, referring to anti-maskers or their behaviours deviating from social norms. "Idiot" was synonymous with anti-maskers in this thread. Positive lexical items such as "good," "great," "proud," and "happy" were used to amplify positive attributes of pro-maskers. Therefore, the A-forum can be characterised as a forum of community building. The thread is also characterised as of high impact but short lifespan. It attracted over 750 posts within a few days, then became inactive quickly and was archived. The thread was dominated by pro-maskers, and it contributed to their sense of community and achievement.

The J-forum on the other hand had few positive evaluative lexical items. This forum is characterised as being confrontational and polarised between pro- and anti-maskers. Where both participants are equally active in posting, they exchange derogatory address terms, and Japanese politeness norms of elevating the other and denigrating self (Gu, 1990; Ohashi, 2008) are openly flouted. The exchanges of derogatory address terms contribute to the simplistic polarisation of the debate into pro- and anti-mask ideologies. Where pro-mask posters are dominant, they demand a regulation (規制 *kisei*) to mandate mask wearing while referring to non-maskers as *baka* or *aho*. Impoliteness observed in the J-forum can also be attributed to the lack of strict rules and enforcement regarding the use of language and content. According to Nishimura (2019), Japanese discussion forums have their own "community of practice" (Wenger, 1998) and some have strict rules on the use of the language, even requiring the use of *desu/masu* honorific endings, for instance. However, the J-forum has no such policy and participants use *tameguchi* (informal style with plain forms). On the other hand, the A-forum has a strict content policy and rules.

7. Conclusion

The two discussion forums illuminate the stark difference, but in both forums evaluative predicates and address terms play significant roles in forming respective social norms. Both forums show the frequent use of negative evaluative labels for anti-maskers and mask sceptics, highlighting that their behaviour is deviating from perceived social norms. In particular, in the J-forum, frequent occurrences of derogatory address terms and *meiwaku* (nuisance) are hurled at anti-maskers and their behaviour which deviates from the desired social norms.

It is worth noting that the A-forum presents positive community building achieved through a collective narrative of being proud of Melbourne for standing up to COVID-19. This particular repertoire is not found in the J-forum. One possible explanation is that wearing a mask was already the norm in Japan, and thus, it was not something to be proud of or feel good about. Considering the concern expressed in the first post about the increasing number of people not wearing masks in public places in Japan, a return to norms was nothing to be proud of. However, for Melburnians, wearing a mask was a new practice, and though there was the mandatory AU$200 fine, the fact that Melburnians quickly adopted the habit of mask wearing may have created positive ground for a sense of solidarity and achievement.

There are numerous online discussion forums and threads about (non-)mask wearing, and each one of them has specific expectations and emerging social norms which reflect local context in a given time and space. Although the study in this chapter employs a cross-cultural perspective, it does not represent culturally comparable reactions to the same stimulus. Each thread represents a collaborative accomplishment by the participants in each specific context. Evaluative predicates, including adjectives/adjectival nouns, and address terms emerge as frequently occurring lexical items for participants, in both discussion forums, to position/align with or distance themselves from a particular ideology or group of people. There may be many other lexical items and emoticons which function in the same way, and further study is necessary to qualitatively delve into more nuanced stance-taking practices in online discussion forums.

Jun Ohashi is Senior Lecturer, Japanese Studies, University of Melbourne. His research investigates interpersonal pragmatics, (im)politeness, critical discourse analysis, media literacy, and linguistic rituals. He has published a monograph *Thanking and Politeness in Japanese* (Palgrave Macmillan, 2013), and papers in *Journal of Pragmatics*, *Multilingua*, and *Journal of Japanese Studies*.

Notes

[1] There is a jurisdictional difference between Japan and Australia. Melbourne is under the jurisdiction of the Victoria State Government. Japan is a unitary state and its central government governs forty-seven prefectures.

2   Historically, Japan has been influenced by Confucianism especially under the Tokugawa shogu-
     nate (1600–1868), and Confucian education was valued in Kyōiku chokugo (Imperial Rescript on
     Education), which was announced in 1890, and later mandated in the education system of Imperial
     Japan (Borton, 1970). Confucianism became less valued as Westernisation advanced, but it is still
     influential "as a moral and ethical code" (Dollinger, 1988, p. 578).
3   NHK緊急事態宣言1回目の状況 [Kinkyū jitai sengen 1-kai-me no jōkyō] (First declaration of a state of
     emergency) https://www3.nhk.or.jp/news/special/coronavirus/emergency/ (accessed 24 April 2022).
4   Ishiyama (2019, p. 37) explains these phenomena as pragmatic depreciation.

References

Batagelj, Borut, Peter Peer, Vitomir Štruc, and Simon Dobrišek. 2021. "How to correctly detect
    face-masks for COVID-19 from visual information?" *Applied Sciences* 11, no. 5: 2070. https://doi.
    org/10.3390/app11052070.

Borton, Hugh. 1970. *Japan's Modern Century: From Perry to 1970.* New York: Roland Press.

Cabani, Adnane, Karim Hammoudi, Halim Benhabiles, and Mahmoud Melkemi. 2021. "MaskedFace-Net
    – A dataset of correctly/incorrectly masked face images in the context of COVID-19." *Smart Health*
    19: 100144. https://doi.org/10.1016/j.smhl.2020.100144.

Chang, Angela, Peter Johannes Schulz, Sheng Tsung Tu, and Matthew Tingchi Liu. 2020. "Commu-
    nicative blame in online communication of the COVID-19 pandemic: Computational approach of
    stigmatizing cues and negative sentiment gauged with automated analytic techniques." *Journal of
    Medical Internet Research* 22, no. 11. https://doi.org/10.2196/21504.

Daijirin. 2006. 3rd ed. Tokyo: Sanseido.

Dollinger, Marc J. 1988. "Confucian ethics and Japanese management practices." *Journal of Business
    Ethics* 7, no. 8: 575–584. https://doi.org/10.1007/bf00382789.

Du Bois, John W. 2007. "The stance triangle." In *Stancetaking in Discourse Subjectivity, Evaluation, Inter-
    action,* edited by Robert Englebretson, 139–182. Amsterdam: John Benjamins Publishing Company.

Elster, Jon. 1989. "Social norms and economic theory." *Journal of Economic Perspectives* 3, no. 4: 99–117.
    https://doi.org/10.1257/jep.3.4.99.

Goffman, Erving. 1967. *Interaction Ritual.* New York: Pantheon.

Gogen Yurai Jiten. [Gogen Yurai Dictionary]. n.d. Accessed September 19, 2021. https://gogen-yurai.jp/.

Gu, Yueguo. 1990. "Politeness phenomena in Modern Chinese." *Journal of Pragmatics* 14, no. 2: 237–257.
    https://doi.org/10.1016/0378-2166(90)90082-0.

Henley, Jon, and Caelainn Barr. 2020. "Global survey shows widespread disapproval of covid response."
    The Guardian, October 27, 2020. https://www.theguardian.com/world/2020/oct/27/global-sur-
    vey-shows-widespread-disapproval-of-covid-response.

Imperial College London. 2020. "COVID-19 behaviour tracker." https://www.imperial.ac.uk/glob-
    al-health-innovation/what-we-do/our-response-to-covid-19/covid-19-behaviour-tracker.

Inglis, David, and Anna-Mari Almila. (2020). "Un-masking the mask: Developing the sociology of facial
    politics in pandemic times and after." *Società Mutamento Politica* 11, no. 21: 251–257. https://doi.
    org/10.13128/smp-11964.

Ishiyama, Osamu. 2019. *Diachrony of Personal Pronouns in Japanese: A Functional and Cross-Linguistic
    Perspective.* Amsterdam: John Benjamins Publishing Company.

Ji, Pan. 2020. "Masking morality in the making: How China's anti-epidemic promotional videos present facemask as a techno-moral mediator." *Social Semiotics* 33, no. 1: 232–239. https://doi.org/10.1080/10350330.2020.1810462.

Kádár, Dániel Z., and Michael Haugh. 2013. *Understanding Politeness.* Cambridge: Cambridge University Press. https://doi.org/10.1017/CBO9781139382717.

Markus, Hazel R., and Shinobu Kitayama. 1991. "Culture and the self: Implications for cognition, emotion, and motivation." *Psychological Review* 98, no. 2: 224–253. https://doi.org/10.1037/0033-295X.98.2.224.

Martin, J. R. 2004. "Mourning: How we get aligned." *Discourse & Society* 15, no. 2–3: 321–344. https://doi.org/10.1177/0957926504041022.

Myers, Greg. 2010. "Stance-taking and public discussion in blogs." *Critical Discourse Studies* 7, no. 4: 263–275. https://doi.org/10.1080/17405904.2010.511832.

Nakayachi, Kazuya, Taku Ozaki, Yukihide Shibata, and Ryosuke Yokoi. 2020. "Why do Japanese people use masks against COVID-19, even though masks are unlikely to offer protection from infection?" *Frontiers in Psychology* 11. https://doi.org/10.3389/fpsyg.2020.01918.

NHK. n.d. "Kinkyū jitai sengen 1-kai-me no jōkyō" [First declaration of a state of emergency]. Accessed April 24, 2022 https://www3.nhk.or.jp/news/special/coronavirus/emergency/.

Nihon Dai Hyakka Zensho [Encyclopaedia of Japan]. 1994. Vol.18. 2nd ed. Tokyo: Shougakukan, 1994.

Ohashi, Jun. 2008. "Linguistic rituals for thanking in Japanese: Balancing obligations." *Journal of Pragmatics* 40, no. 12: 2150–2174. https://doi.org/10.1016/j.pragma.2008.04.001.

Ohashi, Jun. 2021. "#MaskUp in Australia: How social norms in a pandemic are formed." *Melbourne Asia Review.* https://melbourneasiareview.edu.au/maskup-in-australia-how-social-norms-in-a-pandemic-are-formed.

Rich, Motoko, and Hisako Ueno. 2020. "Japan's virus success has puzzled the world: Is its luck running out?" *The New York Times*, March 26, 2020. https://www.nytimes.com/2020/03/26/world/asia/japan-coronavirus.html –commentsContainer.

Sakakibara, Ryota, and Hiroki Ozono. 2020. "Psychological research on the COVID-19 crisis in Japan: Focusing on infection preventive behaviors, future prospects, and information dissemination behaviors." *PsyArXiv* https://doi.org/10.31234/osf.io/635zk [Preprint].

Sakakibara, Ryota, and Hiroki Ozono. 2021. "Why do people wear a mask? A replication of previous studies and examination of two research questions in a Japanese sample." *The Japanese Journal of Psychology* 92, no. 5: 332–338. https://doi.org/10.4992/jjpsy.92.20323

Singelis, Theodore M. 1994. "The measurement of independent and interdependent self-construals." *Personality and Social Psychology Bulletin* 20, no. 5: 580–591. https://doi.org/10.1177/0146167294205014.

Steentjes, Katharine, Tim Kurz, Manuela Barreto, and Thomas A. Morton. 2017. "The norms associated with climate change: Understanding social norms through acts of interpersonal activism." *Global Environmental Change* 43: 116–125. https://doi.org/10.1016/j.gloenvcha.2017.01.008.

Super Daijirin. 2020. Tokyo: Sanseidō.

Suzuki, Takao. 1978. *Japanese and the Japanese: Words in Culture.* Tokyo: Kodansha. [Originally published in Japanese in 1973 as *Kotoba to Bunka*, Tokyo: Iwanami Shoten].

Tajfel, Henri, and John C. Turner. 1986. "The social identity theory of intergroup behavior." In *Psychology of Intergroup Relations*, edited by S. Worchel and W. Austin, 7–24. IL: Nelson-Hall.

The Japan Times. 2020. "Japan's low virus deaths reflect high 'cultural standards,' says Taro Aso." June 5, 2020. https://www.japantimes.co.jp/news/2020/06/05/national/japan-low-virus-deaths-high-cultural-standard-aso/.

Tsukimoro, Osamu. 2021. "With variants on the rise, Japan sticks to firm COVID-19 guidance." *The Japan Times*, July 6, 2021. https://www.japantimes.co.jp/news/2021/07/06/national/variants-japan-corona-virus-guidance/.

Turner, John C., Michael A. Hogg, Penelope J. Oakes, Stephen D. Reicher, and Margaret S. Wetherell. 1987. *Rediscovering the Social Group: A Self-Categorization Theory*. Oxford, UK: Blackwell.

Watts, Richard J. 2003. *Politeness*. Key Topics in Sociolinguistics. Cambridge: Cambridge University Press. https://doi.org/10.1017/CBO9780511615184.

Wenger, Etienne.1998. *Communities of Practice: Learning, Meaning, and Identity*. New York: Cambridge University Press.

Wingfield-Hayes, Rupert. 2020. "Coronavirus: Japan's mysteriously low virus death rate." *BBC News*, July 4, 2020. https://www.bbc.com/news/world-asia-53188847.

CHAPTER 7

COVID-19 and the Construction of Wuli (We): Marriage-Migrant Women and Care Discourses in South Korea

Mi Yung Park & Hakyoon Lee

Abstract

The authors discuss from a critical perspective how bilingual and bicultural capacities of marginalised women in minority groups in South Korea give them agency in contributing to public health initiatives. It is argued that the women's contribution amidst the nation's struggles with COVID-19 has impacted upon the discourse of identity politics.

Keywords: Marriage-migrants, construction of wuli (we), media discourses, bilingual workers, care discourses, identity politics

1. Introduction

South Korea (hereafter "Korea") was one of the first countries affected by COVID-19, reporting its first case on January 20, 2020, when a thermal scanner detected fever in an arrival from China at Incheon International Airport. By September 7, 2021, 220,563,227 cases and 4,565,483 deaths had been reported worldwide (World Health Organization, 2021). In response to the rapid rise in cases early in the pandemic, the Korean government took decisive action by establishing and maintaining approximately six hundred screening and testing centres and adopting strict quarantine policies and a rigorous contact-tracing programme, which tracks infected individuals' previous movements and identifies paths of COVID-19 transmission. Through these strategies, Korea has been able to slow the spread of the virus and keep mortality relatively low.

As a way to increase the efficiency of these measures and practices, the government has actively communicated COVID-19-related information to its citizens, including information on new cases, their sources, and the travel history of confirmed cases. Acknowledging that Korea has become a multicultural and multilingual society, the government has been attempting to provide public health resources in different languages on posters or interpreting and translation services to reach the country's immigrants and foreign workers. In late March 2020, the Government of South Korea launched English and Chinese versions of its official COVID-19 website. However, over a year later, the website had yet to be translated into any other language. Many non-Korean-speaking residents have been unable to access the latest and most accurate information on the pandemic, a challenge also faced by many other linguistic minorities worldwide (Jang and Choi, 2020; Piller, Zhang, and Li, 2020).

Simultaneously, since the COVID-19 outbreak, the treatment of immigrants in Korea has become a serious social and political issue. Korean discrimination against immigrants is not a new phenomenon, but has at times been exacerbated by the Korean government's COVID-19 response. Government policies to mitigate the socioeconomic consequences of COVID-19 have been based on nationality and this in-group/out-group differentiation has resulted in the exclusion of foreign nationals residing in Korea regardless of their legal standing (Lee, Cho, and Jung, 2021). In addition, after a number of infection clusters emerged in Korea's most populous province, Gyeonggi, the government ordered all foreigners and migrant workers residing in the area to get tested, leading to accusations of racial discrimination. The media has also reported that both Koreans and foreign nationals residing in Korea have experienced various types of prejudice in relation to the ongoing public health crisis. Against this background, this chapter brings attention to the ways in which the COVID-19 outbreak caused severe disruption to the lives of marriage-migrant women and investigates how they are perceived and positioned in Korean social discourses related to the disease. COVID-19 affected these women's jobs, language learning, and self-development, as well as their psychological well-being due to social exclusion and reduced ability to visit family back home.

Much of the emphasis in studies of pandemic-related discourses thus far has been on public health, policymaking, and individual hygiene, with little attention to the intersections of these matters with social marginalisation. Therefore, in this study, employing critical discourse analysis, we look at how marriage-migrants' identities and the disruption of their lives are constructed in discourses of care in relation to COVID-19 in the media.

1.1. Background: Discourses of "Multicultural Families" and Marriage-Migrants in Korea

In 2006, the Korean government announced that the nation was in a state of 다문화 사회 [*tamwunhwa sahoy*] (multicultural, multiethnic society) following a rapid increase in the number of immigrants to Korea (Kim, 2011). In particular, Korea has seen a dramatic rise in international marriages, often between foreign women and

Korean men, most of which are facilitated by marriage brokers (Kim, 2008, 2010; Lee, 2014). The influx of female marriage-migrants led the government to create a new family model called the 다문화 가정 [*tamwunhwa kaceng*] (multicultural family), defined as a family with one Korean national spouse and one foreign spouse. The government services and welfare programmes for "multicultural families" are offered exclusively to these families; they exclude migrants who are not married to Korean nationals, such as foreign workers who reside in Korea (Kim, 2016). Women who are marriage-migrants are viewed as potential Korean citizens, given their role in the biological and cultural reproduction of the nation. Accordingly, the government's policies and social integration programmes for these women fall within a "patriarchal family-oriented welfare model," in which the main aim is to enable foreign brides to successfully manage family- and household-making (Kim, 2011; Lee, 2014).

In public discourses, migrant women are typically positioned as racialised, gendered "others" with inadequate cultural capital who need to be acculturated into Korean society. First, the government tends to construct the women as "unskilled mothers" who may have difficulty raising and educating their children (Bélanger, Lee, and Wang, 2010). Much is made of the women's lack of Korean language and cultural knowledge and the impact this will have on the next generation. Second, the nature of their migration evokes two seemingly opposite stereotypes: foreign brides as "vulnerable victims of a male-operated international trade," or, more commonly, "manipulative opportunists who marry solely for economic security" (Kim, 2010, p. 718). The latter image of foreign brides has become widespread partly due to media portrayals of migration-related marriage fraud (Freeman, 2011). This view has also created an image of the women as potential "runaways," who marry Koreans only to earn money to support their families back home, and feel no obligation to stay with their Korean spouses (Freeman, 2011). These existing discourses and stereotypes generated in the host society contribute to the struggles faced by the migrants as they strive to adapt and construct meaningful identities in their new homes. Research on the postmigration experiences of marriage-migrants in Korea has demonstrated the difficulties they experience in fully integrating into Korean society and in preserving their cultures and identities related to their countries of origin (Freeman, 2011; Hong, Song, and Park, 2013; Kim, 2008, 2010; Park, 2017, 2019, 2020; Schubert, Lee, and Lee, 2015).

The Korean government has acknowledged the linguistic and cultural resources which marriage-migrants bring to the country, as reflected in the Basic Plan for Multicultural Family Policies (Ministry of Gender Equality and Family, 2018). The government has tried to cultivate marriage-migrants as a human resource, in part by transforming them from "Korean language learners" into "bilingual workers," such as multicultural instructors and interpreters (Sohn and Kang, 2021).

By validating the bilingual competencies of the migrant women, the government has also tried to foster bilingualism for their children, positioning the children as global resources for the nation due to their potential linguistic and cultural capital (Shin, 2019). The positioning of marriage-migrants and multicultural families—by the government, the media, mainstream society, and themselves—is complex and multifaceted. Within the discourse of human capital, differences in linguistic and cultural backgrounds which are often used to marginalise migrant women and their children are instead reframed as an asset for the society.

1.2 The Discursive Construction of Wuli (We)

우리 [wuli] (we) is a Korean first-person plural pronoun meaning we/our. As with the English we, it can be inclusive or exclusive. Its meaning is fluid, as its referent can have multiple and changing memberships, which are always determined by the sociolinguistic and interactional context in which the word is uttered (Helmbrecht, 2002; Mühlhäusler and Harré, 1990; Pavlidou, 2014; Song, 2019). While a few previous studies have examined wuli (e.g., Kim, 2009; Lee, 2020; Lim, 2018; Song, 2019), it has not been much discussed in terms of social discourse. An important feature of Korean wuli is that it can be used inclusively, and be more felicitous than a singular pronoun, even when the addressee is not literally included in the specific context, in which case its use has to do with the social relationship of the speaker and addressee e.g., 우리 남편 [wuli nampyen] (our husband) in a non-polygamous context (Kim et al., 2003; Song, 2019, pp. 13–14).

There have been various analyses of wuli presented in the literature. Some scholars have claimed that this aspect of wuli reflects the "collectivist" culture of Korea (or East Asia generally, in contrast to Western "individualist" cultures; Hofstede, 1991). Song (2019) suggested more particularly that wuli can be used to evoke a "Korean-specific personhood that emphasises intersubjectivities among group members" (p. 18). Kim (2009), comparing the English and Korean use of the second- and first-person plural pronouns in popular science texts, attributed the observed quantitative and qualitative differences to sociocultural influences. For example, a collectivistic tendency in Korean society could lead to a general preference for wuli over 당신 [tangsin] (you), because the second-person pronoun evokes a sense of one individual being singled out.

Lee (2015), who used a corpus-based approach, discussed a variety of nonindexical or non-deictic functions of wuli, including as a stance marker which can express the speaker's affection. Other scholars have investigated the pragmatic meanings of wuli. Lee (2020), for instance, discussed how the two first-person possessive pronouns, 내 [nay] (my) and wuli, are used to express distinct connotations, with wuli conveying group belonging, affection, or generality. Lim (2018) also claims that *wuli* not only refers to normal plurality, but has special uses and meanings, such as showing solidarity with hearers or presenting opinions as if they are objective.

Another body of research has focused on the linguistic meanings of *wuli* versus *nay* "my/me" as contrastive notions. For example, Yoon (2003) argues that *wuli* is an in-group membership marker rather than the plural form of *nay*, and that age and gender are crucial factors in selecting either *wuli* or *nay*. According to Lee (2007), the use of *wuli* instead of *nay* implies the primary familial bonds of Korean culture. In this study, we examine *wuli* as a cultural (Na and Choi, 2009) or ideological construct, rather than linguistic. Thus, instead of examining the linguistic meaning of *wuli* in the data, we consider how the inclusive or exclusive contrast is constructed in the data as a type of metaphor for social exclusion in a collectivist society.

2. The Study

2.1 Critical Discourse Analysis

In Critical Discourse Analysis (CDA), language is viewed as a social practice. Critically analysing how language is used is considered a means of empowering individuals and social groups. CDA has been applied to mass-media discourses (Abdullah, 2014; Molina, 2009; Sari et al., 2018), often as a tool to explore socio-political issues and understand how ideologies and public discourses affect each other. For example, using CDA as an analytic tool, Song (2013) demonstrates reproduction of unequal power relationships between cultures and languages in a Korean English-education television programme where American English is portrayed as the preferred variety of English. Lee (2019) used a text-mining approach to investigate the representation of immigrant workers in Korean news reporting and showed that Koreans were represented as "us," implying Korea is a homogeneous country. In this study, we apply CDA to Korean media discourses of multicultural families and marriage-migrants during the COVID-19 pandemic, focusing on how linguistic and cultural ideologies are used to socially position particular groups in such discourses.

In the Korean context, previous CDA studies have focused on how different populations or social issues are depicted in media. For example, topics such as bullying in schools (Park, 2004), the abolition of the National Security Laws (Lee, 2005), and individualism in Korean society (Kuk and Jang, 2011) have all been investigated. In a more recent CDA study, Kim and Yoo (2019) analysed newspaper articles to examine a phenomenon known as 맘충 [*mamchwung*] (lit. mom-roach), a newly coined and derogatory internet word used to describe mothers who never punish their children. Another recent CDA study on Korean media was conducted by Ahn

(2018), who investigated media representations of the trend of 농촌 유학 [*nongchon yuhak*] (schooling in farm villages).

A few other studies have critically examined how multicultural families are described in the Korean media. Hwang (2017) analysed anti-multicultural discourses, Park (2013) examined anti- and pro-multiculturalism online, Shin (2019) focused on multicultural children and their portrayal in newspapers, and Suh and Kim (2019) explored how Southeast Asian immigrants in Korea were represented in the media. Similarly, Joo's (2012) study on representations of migrants in Korean public broadcasting news showed the discursive construction of discrimination in Korean media where immigrants are depicted as "others." Chung et al. (2021) conducted an inductive framing analysis during the COVID-19 pandemic and observed the political and social construction of national or racialised "others" in the media. The study in this chapter contributes to the growing discussion on multicultural families and marriage-migrants by examining media representations of marriage-migrants in relation to COVID-19 and discourses of care from a CDA perspective. In the following section, we describe how we collected and analysed the data for this study.

2.2 Data and Analysis

The study examines forty-two articles published during the pandemic by diverse Korean news sources. Using internet browsers, we searched for news articles originally published either online or offline between March 1, 2020 and May 31, 2021 and containing any of a set of key words and phrases (e.g., "multicultural families," "COVID-19," "bilingual families," "multicultural centre," and 마음 방역 [*maum pangyek*] (prevention of mental illness)). The two authors first analysed each article separately, focusing on how multicultural families or marriage-migrant women were positioned in the article. After this individual analysis, the authors shared their preliminary findings, and then worked together to find common themes and organise the data into categories.

Two broadly salient themes emerged from the initial analysis: inclusivity and exclusivity. Of the 42 articles collected, 25 are based on inclusive discourses and 17 on exclusive discourses. We would like to note that most articles were from local newspapers whose primary audience is the residents of rural areas.

In the following section, we discuss our findings on the two contrastive discourses around multicultural families and marriage-migrants and the pandemic: exclusive discourses which position multicultural families and marriage-migrants as outsiders or "others," and inclusive discourses which position them as insiders by depicting them as key members of society.

3. Findings

3.1 Discourses of Exclusivity: Constructing Marriage-Migrants as "Others"

The most prevalent discourses about multicultural families and marriage-migrant women emphasise marriage-migrants' marginal status in the society and the challenges they face on account of their (perceived) lack of language proficiency, as well as their gender and socioeconomic status. As mentioned in the introduction, their position is often reinforced in COVID-19-related discourses as foreigners who are less likely to possess advanced Korean language skills and whose access to resources is restricted. The media examples we present illustrate how restrictive measures during COVID-19 infection waves caused major disruption to migrant women's work and lives, as well as illustrate their inability to manage this *disruption.*

On March 9, 2021, *Yenhap News* reported on the findings of a research project conducted by Dongguk University's Institute for Multicultural Integration, which examined news articles mentioning the word "multicultural" before and during the COVID-19 pandemic (2019–2020). The study analysed approximately 4,000 articles published in fifty-four major media outlets, including newspapers, in Korea. It found that in references to multicultural issues, positive words, such as "interest," "fondness," and "joyfulness" had decreased since the pandemic began, while negative words, such as "resistance," "fear," and "sadness" had noticeably increased. In addition, words referring to positive interactions amongst people and groups, including "communication" and "understanding" had also decreased.

During the pandemic, much attention has been directed towards individual hygiene and physical health, but health and hygiene discourses around particular groups and group cultures have also emerged. On March 21, 2021, for example, *Pyeonghwa News*, an online newspaper based in Gyeongbuk province, reported on discrimination against migrant workers regarding the COVID-19 test. According to the article, the city of Daegu implemented particularly intense COVID-19 testing policies specifically for migrant factory workers. Various citizen organisations and human rights groups protested against this unequal implementation of testing policies as discriminatory.

Discourses of the marginalisation of multicultural families and marriage-migrants became stronger as the media highlighted the isolation of migrants in the pandemic. For instance, some media focused on COVID-19's particularly severe disruption of marriage-migrant women's lives, as it created obstacles to their language learning or self-development.

A news article in *Hankook Ilbo* entitled 코로나19가 높인 언어 장벽 ... 이주 여성의 고군분투 "한국어 배우기" [*kholona 19ka nophin ene cangpyek ... icwu yesenguy kokwunpwunthwu "hankwuke paywuki"*] (Language Barriers Exacerbated by COVID-19

... Migrant Women's Struggle to Learn Korean) paints a vivid image of marriage-migrants' lack of Korean proficiency. It describes how this problem has been exacerbated by the suspension of face-to-face Korean language instruction, due to the four-month closure of the Multicultural Family Support Centres during the COVID-19 pandemic. The excerpt below details an interview with two marriage-migrant women who described the problems they faced due to the cancellation of classes:

> One lady, who has lived in Korea for eight years, said, "I forgot a lot of Korean during the three months when classes weren't offered." Another person, who has lived in Korea for 12 years, said, "I need to know not only how to speak, but also how to write and read, so that I can help my children study Korean at home, but I was frustrated because I couldn't." As parents of Korea-born children, it is not easy for them to cope with the stress associated with language barriers. (Taewoong Lee and Haein Lee, May 31, 2020)

By highlighting language barriers despite the women's long residence in Korea, and positing their lack of Korean proficiency as the main reason they struggled to educate their children, the article positions them as unskilled foreign mothers. In particular, the article emphasises migrant women's lack of Korean literacy as a unique manifestation of the general frustration of parenting during the pandemic, making it a factor which divides "us" from "them."

In addition, while the article describes the implementation of online classes as 가뭄의 단비 [kamwumuy tanpi] (a welcoming rain in the drought) for marriage-migrants, it also depicts online instruction in largely negative terms, mainly due to the women's poverty and assumed role as their children's primary caregivers, both of which limit their ability to benefit from online instruction at home, as shown below:

> A Vietnamese woman who migrated to Korea in 2012 has to work at a cafe on weekdays ... [but also] has to take care of her children who are unable to go to school due to COVID-19. She said, "Before COVID-19, childcare classes were held at the same time as my Korean classes at the Multicultural Education Centre, so I could leave my children there while attending classes." However, after childcare classes were suspended due to COVID-19, migrant women had no choice but to attend classes online while taking care of their children at home. (Taewoong Lee and Haein Lee, May 31, 2020)

Another interviewee was quoted as saying, "I couldn't concentrate on my studies at home [when] my child was saying, 'Mom, what are you doing? Play with me!'" This article underscores a perception that migrant mothers' primary purpose is to be caregivers, in addition to emphasising the problems they encountered in accessing learning opportunities at home and the deterioration of their Korean skills due to the cancellation of classes caused by COVID-19.

Significantly reduced mobility and staying home during the pandemic has also contributed to increased domestic violence. One article from online news source *News1*, entitled 코로나19로 악화?... "다문화 가정폭력 도와주세요" [*kholona 19lo akhwa?... "tamwunhwa kacengphoklyek towacwuseyyo"*] (Worse with COVID-19? "Please Help Stop Domestic Violence in Multicultural Families"), attributed conflicts in multicultural families largely to language barriers:

> Some migrant women are vulnerable to domestic violence so support measures are needed. Communication problems are at the root of the conflict, and due to COVID-19, the whole family is gathered in one house. Thus, marital problems become magnified because they are taking their personal stresses out on each other. (Harim Park, June 19, 2020)

Although domestic violence and marital problems have increased in many families during the pandemic, media discourses which focus on migrants have largely depicted these problems as the result of a language barrier and therefore unique to multicultural families. This perception is again based on an "us" versus "them" mindset, and it reinforces the idea that some of the negative impacts of the pandemic only affect migrant families.

In addition, positioning the women as linguistically incompetent, the article problematises their lack of proficiency in Korean as the "root" cause of the increase in domestic violence:

> Most migrant women do not have the Korean language ability to completely resolve misunderstandings arising from such situations through dialogue. In the end, some men who lack patience cannot solve problems through conversation and end up using domestic violence. (Harim Park, June 19, 2020)

The article also highlights the migrant women's helplessness due to their financial situation:

> When confronted with extreme domestic violence by a spouse, the Police and the Multicultural Family Centre work together to actively respond. However, many immigrant women who have immigrated to Korea due to their family's financial hardship try to cope with the problem themselves in order to send money to their families back home. When such problems are repeated and when they hit a wall, it is often the case that multicultural couples end up getting a divorce. (Harim Park, June 19, 2020)

The neediness of their birth families, whose socioeconomic status is assumed to be low, is given as the reason these women hesitate to seek help when they face domestic violence. The article then suggests that the women's failure to cope on their own may lead to family breakup. By portraying migrant women's situations as being exacerbated by their lack of Korean language proficiency and their financial difficulties, and not by the imposition of COVID-19 closures, this article creates the idea that "we as Koreans" have the upper hand in self-sufficiency, reinforcing the notion of migrant women as "others."

In addition, even though everybody experienced travel restrictions and reduced social interactions due to the pandemic, the media often portrayed migrants as suffering particularly from social isolation and their inability to go "back home" to their country of origin. The article 고향 못가는 다문화가족, 용기 갖고 희망의 봄 기다리 길 [*kohyang moskanun tamwunhwakacok, yongki kacko huymanguy pom kitalikil*] (Multicultural Families Unable to Go Home Due to COVID-19: Wait and Hope), in *Gyeonggi Multicultural Family News*, depicts marriage-migrant women as "people who cannot go home," "those who can't help but spend New Year's Day lonely," and people "who suffer more due to their migration background" (Haseong Song, February 24, 2021). Although this article employs a sympathetic frame, it positions the women as helpless foreigners with distant families, rather than as Korean citizens with immediate family in Korea, while emphasising their distance from "home" as the cause of their suffering and loneliness during the pandemic.

Overall, these news articles position migrant women as unskilled foreign-born mothers of Korean-born children, and stress their isolated, powerless, and vulnerable situation due to the social isolation resulting from the COVID-19 pandemic. In these articles, which address issues of gender, language, and domestic violence, the use of expressions which exclude the migrant women from membership in mainstream Korean society, such as 외국인 결혼 이주 여성 [*oykwukin kyelhon icwu yeseng*] (foreign marriage-migrant women), 외국서 결혼이주해 온 여성 [*oykwukse kyelhonicwuhay on yeseng*] (women who migrated from a foreign country), 결혼 이 주민 [*kyelhon icwumin*] (marriage-migrants), and 이주 여성 [*icwu yeseng*] (immigrant women), contributes to constructing the women as "other" and strengthening an in-group culture (*wuli*) to which they are outsiders. In addition, some expressions which describe the migrant women's situation during the pandemic, such as 언 어 장벽 [*ene cangpyek*] (language obstacles), 생존 수단 [*sayngcon swutan*] (survival means), and 방역의 사각지대 [*pangyekuy sakakcitay*] (blind spot of the prevention), highlight and particularise the difficulties they face specifically due to their "otherness."

In the next section, we discuss how the media contrastively constructs and uses inclusive discourses as a strategy to reframe migrant women as valuable bilingual citizens who can be useful for effectively responding to the COVID-19 crisis.

3.2 Discourses of Inclusivity: Reframing Marriage-Migrants as Valuable Bilingual Citizens

In contrast to the discourses of exclusivity which position marriage-migrants as incompetent and marginalised, a discourse of marriage-migrants as human capital characterises them as offering a cultural and linguistic bridge between mainstream Korean society and the marriage-migrants' co-ethnic foreign residents, and thus a useful resource for responding to the COVID-19 pandemic. In this section, we discuss how the cultural and linguistic backgrounds which distinguish these women from monolingual and monocultural Koreans are reframed as valuable resources for effective cross-cultural communication in the context of emergency preparedness and response.

For instance, one news report from *Gyeonggi Sisa Today*, entitled 다문화가족 통역지원단, 이천시와 발맞춰 코로나 대응에 힘써 [*tamwunhwakacok thongyekciwentan, ichensiwa palmacchwe kholona tayungey himsse*] (Interpretation Support Group for Multicultural Families: Responding to COVID-19 in Step with Icheon City), summarised the situation as follows:

> In cooperation with the Interpretation Support Team of the Icheon City's Health, Family, and Multicultural Family Support Centre, the city of Icheon has made a concerted and determined approach to prevent the spread of COVID-19 … sixteen people from China, Cambodia, Vietnam, Japan, Philippines, Russia, Mongolia, Thailand, and Myanmar are currently providing interpretation and translation services in nine different languages. (Haneul Kim, April 13, 2020)

An article from *Dong-a Ilbo*, entitled 대구 결혼이주여성들도 코로나 방역 동참 [*taykwu kyelhonicwuyesengtulto kholona pangyek tongcham*] (Co-participation of Marriage-Migrant Women from Daegu in COVID-19 Prevention), stressed how their interpretation work contributes to the fight against COVID-19. The word "co-participation" in the title implies a collaborative relationship between marriage-migrants and the city, Daegu, the site of Korea's worst COVID-19 outbreak to date. The report described the women's role as follows:

> In particular, it is difficult to closely manage foreigners due to language barriers during self-quarantine. In Daegu, as of 29 June 2020, there are 161 foreigners in self-isolation. Marriage-migrant women who belong to the Support Centre for Health, Households, and Multicultural Families formed an interpreting service team to support monitoring of foreigners in self-isolation. Eighty-six marriage-migrants from nine countries took care of 860 foreigners from 8 April 2020 to 30 June 2020. (Minjun Myung, June 30, 2020)

In this article, marriage-migrant women are portrayed as exerting an important and powerful influence on the management of foreigners in quarantine by serving as information mediators and overcoming language barriers, as highlighted in the large number of foreigners they assisted. By framing their service as "cooperation" or "collaboration," this article presents marriage-migrant women as socially responsible and "good" citizens. This aligns with the construction of a more inclusive national discourse of *"wuli"* by treating them as participants in Korean society's sharing of "intersubjectivities among group members" (Song, 2019, p. 18).

The article also offers the following quote from an interview with the manager of Daegu's Department of Family and Women Policies, which depicts marriage-migrant women as enabling the city to support foreigners in quarantine:

> It was expected that it would be difficult to take care of foreigners in self-quarantine, but the city is coping with the COVID-19 situation well because marriage-migrant women have been helping. We plan to share this widely as a good strategy for overcoming COVID-19. (Minjun Myung, June 30, 2020)

Acknowledging the challenges arising from language barriers in terms of disseminating COVID-19-related information and supporting foreigners, the article stresses the utilisation of marriage-migrants' linguistic resources as an effective way to overcome these challenges and provide foreigners with equitable access to information.

Other newspaper articles show how marriage-migrants serve as safety and health care providers who help foreigners access health care information and services, strengthening the discourse of marriage-migrants as human resources due to their multilingual and multicultural skills. An article in *Siheung Journal*, entitled 결혼 이주여성 안전보건강사 "마음 방역 톡톡" [*kyelhonicwuyeseng ancenpokenkangsa "maum pangyek thokthok"*] (Female Marriage-Migrants as Safety and Health Care Instructors: "Prevention of Mental Illness"), offers a vivid example of their activities in Siheung, where over ten per cent of the population of the city are foreign residents: "Siheung City's Jeongwang Health Centre cooperates with marriage-migrant women who are safety and health care providers to offer foreigners thorough COVID-19–related consultation, including test guidelines and self-quarantine rules" (Jongseok Byun, March 10, 2021). The article highlights the importance of their work for the mental health of foreign residents as well as their physical health, as in the following excerpt:

> A foreign resident who used the screening clinic stated, "Given language barriers and COVID-19 anxiety, getting assistance in my own native language helped me feel at ease." We plan to continue fostering safety and health care providers in order to ensure foreign employees' mental health and create healthy and safe workplaces. (Jongseok Byun, March 10, 2021)

Linking shared language and adequate understanding to mental well-being, this article suggests marriage-migrants' potential to contribute to the management of COVID-19 and mental health support for foreign residents by bringing a level of ease and comfort to these interactions.

In the discourse of marriage-migrants as human capital, their linguistic and cultural resources are categorised as an asset to Korea in the state of emergency caused by the pandemic. To emphasise how they are playing their part as members of Korean society to help prevent the spread of COVID-19, the articles use words and phrases such as 힘을 보태다 [*himul pothayta*] (add strength), 발을 맞추다 [*palul macchwuta*] (to be in step with), 동참 [*tongcham*] (co-participation), and 협력 [*hye-plyek*] (cooperation), highlighting collective responsibility and partnership, and perhaps contributing to a shift in the discourses of *"wuli."* By discursively positioning marriage-migrants as active "co-participants" in helping to fight against and overcome disruptions caused by COVID-19, and hence insiders, these reports may help build a more united society in Korea, while also generating and strengthening a discourse in which *wuli* includes both Koreans and (some) migrants.

Conclusion

The COVID-19 pandemic has caused extraordinary disruptions to everyday life. This study investigated coexisting and contrastive media discourses around marriage-migrants in Korea in this context of disruption and emergency. By critically analysing articles from diverse media sources, this study showed how two distinct social discourses were produced and reinforced to position the marriage-migrants as socially "other" and at the same time to reframe them as bilingual resources. They are described as powerless, less competent, and disadvantaged foreigners whose lives were immensely disrupted and affected by the pandemic. On the other hand, they are also depicted as powerful because they are competent bilingual resources who can bridge the gap between non-Korean residents of Korea and mainstream Korean society. Somewhat ironically, they are portrayed as vulnerable and incapable of educating their children due to a lack of Korean proficiency even as their bilingual abilities make them valuable members of society who can help fight the spread of disease.

The findings of this study demonstrate that multiple linguistic and cultural ideologies around migrant women coexist and are reproduced and reinforced in media. Two broadly contrastive ideas—which can be articulated as exclusive *wuli* and inclusive *wuli*—are both strategically constructed as fitting within the pursuit of social harmony amongst "us Koreans." Worldwide, as the pandemic continues, discourses of blame criticising migrants and travellers as causing the global pandemic may further shift towards discourses of cooperation which emphasise shared social responsibility, the value of bilingual ability in times of crisis, and the inclusive construction of who counts as "we."

This study examines how a local landscape has been affected by the global pandemic through the lens of critical media analysis. Linguistically, some key expressions emerged as evidence of both exclusive discourses, such as 언어 장벽 [*ene cangpyek*] (language obstacles), 생존 수단 [*sayngcon swutan*] (means of survival), and 방역의 사각지대 [*pangyekuy sakakcitay*] (blind spot of prevention), and inclusive discourses, such as 힘을 보태다 [*himul pothayta*] (add strength), 발을 맞추다 [*palul macchwuta*] (to be in step with), 동참 [*tongcham*] (co-participation), and 협력 [*hyeplyek*] (cooperation).

Korea's responses to COVID-19 reveal how collective responsibility and care are co-constructed by states and citizens, locally and nationally, in the midst of disruption. The notion of immigrants as "others" is reinforced by discourses centred around isolating outsiders as an apparent threat, while it is challenged by discourses focused on the goal of uniting the society by expanding the definition of an insider.

Mi Yung Park is Senior Lecturer in Korean at the University of Auckland. Her research interests include sociolinguistics, heritage language maintenance, and language and identity. Her work has appeared in journals such as *International Journal of Bilingual Education and Bilingualism*, *Language and Intercultural Communication*, *Language Awareness*, and *Journal of Pragmatics*.

Hakyoon Lee is Associate Professor of Korean, Department of World Languages and Cultures, Georgia State University. Hakyoon researches at the intersection of language and identity, sociolinguistics, bilingualism, multilingualism, and immigrant education. Her work has appeared in *Applied Linguistics*, *Applied Linguistics Review*, *Narrative Inquiry*, and *Journal of Language, Identity, and Education*.

References

Abdullah, Faiz Sathi. 2014. "Mass media discourse: A critical analysis research agenda." *Pertanika Journal of Social Science & Humanities* 22: 1–18.

Ahn, Saerom. 2018. "Mitie tamlonulo pon nongchonyuhakuy uymi kwusengkwa silchen" [Discursive practices of schooling in farm villages in media discourses: A critical discourse analysis of the documentary *A Rural School, Urban Children*]. *Hwankyeng Kyoyuk* 31, no. 3: 224–240.

Bélanger, Danièle, Hye-Kyung Lee, and Hong-Zen Wang. 2010. "Ethnic diversity and statistics in East Asia: 'Foreign brides' surveys in Taiwan and South Korea." *Ethnic and Racial Studies* 33, no. 6: 1108–1130.

Byun, Jongseok. 2021. "Female marriage-migrants as safety and health care instructors: 'Prevention of mental illness.'" *Siheung Journal*, March 10, 2021. http://www.shjn.co.kr/news/articleView. html?idxno=60913.

Chung, Angie. Y, Hyerim Jo, Ji-won Lee, and Fan Yang. 2021. "COVID-19 and the political framing of China, nationalism, and borders in the US and South Korean news media." *Sociological Perspectives* 64, no. 5: 747–764.

Freeman, Caren. 2011. *Making and Faking Kinship: Marriage and Labor Migration between China and South Korea*. Ithaca, NY: Cornell University Press.

Helmbrecht, Johannes. 2002. "Grammar and function of *we*." In *Us and Others: Social Identities across Languages, Discourses and Cultures*, edited by Anna Duszak, 31–49. Amsterdam: John Benjamins.

Hofstede, Geert. 1991. *Organization and Culture: Software of the Mind*. New York: McGraw-Hill.

Hong, Yihua, Changzoo Song, and Julie Park. 2013. "Korean, Chinese, or what? Identity transformations of Chosonjok (Korean Chinese) migrant brides in South Korea." *Asian Ethnicity* 14, no. 1: 29–51.

Hwang, Kyongah. 2017. "Pantamwunhwa tamlonuy pwusangkwa enlonuy cayhyen = <cosenilpo>wa <hankyeleysinmwun>uy pantamwunhwa kwanlyen kisaey tayhan theyksuthupwunsekul cwungsimulo" [The paradox of multiculturalism reflected in media discourses: Representation of anti-multicultural sentiments]. *Mitie, Ceynte & Mwunhwa* 32, no. 4: 143–189.

Jang, In Chull, and Lee Jin Choi. 2020. "Staying connected during COVID-19: The social and communicative role of an ethnic online community of Chinese international students in South Korea." *Multilingua* 39, no. 5: 541–552.

Joo, Jaewon. 2012. "The discursive construction of discrimination: The representation of ethnic diversity in the Korean public service broadcasting news." PhD diss., London School of Economics and Political Science.

Kim, Anna. 2016. "Welfare policies and budget allocation for migrants in South Korea." *Asian and Pacific Migration Journal* 25, no. 1: 85–96.

Kim, Chul Kyu. 2009. "Personal pronouns in English and Korean texts: A corpus-based study in terms of textual interaction." *Journal of Pragmatics* 41, no. 10: 2086–2099.

Kim, Haneul. 2020. "Interpretation support group for multicultural families: Responding to COVID-19 in step with Icheon City." *Gyeonggi Sisa Today*, April 13, 2020. https://www.yitoday.com/news/articleView.html?idxno=76101.

Kim, Hyun Mee. 2011. "The emergence of the 'multicultural family' and genderized citizenship in South Korea." In *Contested Citizenship in East Asia: Developmental Politics, National Unity, and Globalization*, edited by Kyung-Sup Chang and Bryan S. Turner, 203–217. New York: Routledge.

Kim, Kil Young, Dong Hwa Kim, Bok Hee Kim, Suk Ja Seong, Hye Kyeong Jang, Yun Jeong Cha, et al. 2003. *Hankwuke hwayonglon* [Korean pragmatics]. Seoul: Sejong.

Kim, Minjeong. 2008. "Gendering marriage emigration and fragmented citizenship formation: 'Korean' wives, daughters-in-law, and mothers from the Philippines." PhD diss., State University of New York, Albany.

Kim, Minjeong. 2010. "Gender and international marriage migration." *Sociology Compass* 4, no. 9: 718–731.

Kim, Yi-Gyeong, and Mee Sook Yoo. 2019. "Mamchwung homyengey tayhan tamlon pwunsek: Kisa pwunsekul cwungsimulo" [Discourse analysis of the use of the term *mamchoong* ("mum-roach"): Focusing on newspaper articles]. *Global Creative Leader: Education & Learning* 9, no. 1: 43–63.

Kuk, Yeong Hi, and Ha Rim Jang. 2011. "Mitietamlon sok mwunhwayuhyengey kwanhan yenkwu – kayincwuuy nonuylul cwungsimulo" [A study of cultural patterns in media discourse: Focusing on the concept of individualism]. *Hankwukcachihayngcenghakpo* 25, no. 2: 177–195.

Lee, Changsoo. 2019. "How are 'immigrant workers' represented in Korean news reporting?—A text mining approach to critical discourse analysis." *Digital Scholarship in the Humanities*, 34, no. 1: 82–99.

Lee, Han-Gyu. 2007. "Hankwuke taymyengsa 'wuli'" [A pragmatic and sociocultural approach to the so-called 1st person pronoun *wuli* in Korean]. *Tamhwawa Inchi* 14, no. 3: 155–178.

Lee, Hye-Kyung. 2014. "The role of multicultural families in South Korean immigration policy." In *Asian Women and Intimate Work*, edited by Emiko Ochiai and Kaoru Aoyama, 289–312. Leiden: Brill.

Lee, Hye-Kyung. 2015. "A corpus-pragmatic analysis of *Wuli*." *Tamhwawa Inchi* 22, no. 3: 59–78.

Lee, Hye-Kyung. 2020. "The use of the Korean first person possessive pronoun *Nay* vis-à-vis *Wuli*." *Language and Linguistics* 21, no. 1: 33–53.

Lee, Juheon, Sarah Cho, and Gowoon Jung. 2021. "Policy responses to COVID-19 and discrimination against foreign nationals in South Korea." *Critical Asian Studies*. https://doi.org/10.1080/14672715 .2021.1897472.

Lee, Taewoong, and Haein Lee. 2020. "Language barriers exacerbated by COVID-19 ... migrant women's struggle to learn Korean." *Hankook Ilbo*. May 13. https://www.hankookilbo.com/News/ Read/202005251739393273.

Lee, Won-Pyo. 2005. "Sinmwun saseleyseuy inyem phyohyeney tayhan enehakcek pwunsek: 'kwukkapoanpep' phyeyciey tayhan noncaynguy kyengwu" [A linguistic analysis of ideologies in newspaper editorials: Focusing on the disputes about the abolition of the "National Security Laws"]. *Sahoyenehak* 13, no. 1: 191–227.

Lim, Donghoon. 2018. "Pragmatic effects of number and person in Korean pronominal system: Three uses of first person plural *Wuli*." *Lingua* 204, (March): 1–15.

Ministry of Gender Equality and Family. 2018. *Cey3cha tamwunhwakacokcengchayk kiponkyeyhoyk (2018–2022)* [The third basic plan for multicultural family policy (2018–2022)]. Seoul, Korea: Ministry of Gender Equality and Family.

Molina, Pedro Santander. 2009. "Critical analysis of discourse and of the media: Challenges and shortcomings." *Critical Discourse Studies* 6, no. 3: 185–198.

Mühlhäusler, Peter, and Ron Harré. 1990. *Pronouns and People*. Cambridge, MA: Blackwell.

Myung, Minjun. 2020. "Co-participation of marriage-migrant women from Daegu in COVID-19 prevention." *Dong-a Ilbo*, June 30, 2020. https://www.donga.com/news/article/all/20200629/101741737/1?comm.

Na, Jinkyung, and Incheol Choi. 2009. "Culture and first-person pronouns." *Personality and Social Psychology Bulletin* 35, no. 11: 1492–1499.

Park, Gil Ja. 2004. "Discourse analysis of school bullying videos." *Korean Journal of Youth Studies* 11, no. 1: 331–360.

Park, Harim. 2020. "Worse with COVID-19? 'Please help stop domestic violence in multicultural families.'" *News1*, June 19. 2020. https://www.news1.kr/articles/?3970163.

Park, Hyu-Yong. 2013. "Critical analysis of contrasting identities and styles of anti- and pro-multicultural discourses in Korea." *Sahoyenehak* 12, no. 3: 157–179.

Park, Mi Yung. 2017. "Resisting linguistic and ethnic marginalization: Voices of Southeast Asian marriage-migrant women in Korea." *Language and Intercultural Communication* 17, no. 2: 118–134.

Park, Mi Yung. 2019. "Challenges of maintaining the mother's language: Marriage-migrants and their mixed-heritage children in South Korea." *Language and Education* 33, no. 5: 431–444.

Park, Mi Yung. 2020. "'I want to learn Seoul speech!': Language ideologies and practices among marriage-migrants in South Korea." *International Journal of Bilingual Education and Bilingualism* 23, no. 2: 227–240.

Pavlidou, Theodossia-Soula. 2014. "Constructing collectivity with 'we': An introduction." In *Constructing Collectivity: "We" across Languages and Contexts*, edited by Theodossia-Soula Pavlidou, 1–22. Amsterdam: John Benjamins.

Piller, Ingrid, Jie Zhang, and Jia Li. 2020. "Linguistic diversity in a time of crisis: Language challenges of the COVID-19 pandemic." *Multilingua* 39, no. 5: 503–515. https://doi.org/10.1515/multi-2020-0136.

Sari, Ratna, Silvia Eka Putri, Herdi, and Budianto Hamuddin. 2018. "Bridging critical discourse analysis in media discourse studies." *Indonesian EFL Journal* 4, no. 2: 80–89.

Schubert, Amelia L., Youngmin Lee, and Hyun-Uk Lee. 2015. "Reproducing hybridity in Korea: Conflicting interpretations of Korean culture by South Koreans and ethnic Korean Chinese marriage migrants." *Asian Journal of Women's Studies* 21, no. 3: 232–251.

Shin, Jaran. 2019. "The vortex of multiculturalism in South Korea: A critical discourse analysis of the characterization of 'multicultural children' in three newspapers." *Communication and Critical/Cultural Studies* 16, no. 1: 61–81. https://doi.org/10.1080/14791420.2019.1590612.

Sohn, Bong-Gi, and Mia Kang. 2021. "'We contribute to the development of South Korea': Bilingual womanhood and politics of bilingual policy in South Korea." *Multilingua* 40, no. 2: 175–198.

Song, Haseong. 2021. "Multicultural families unable to go home due to COVID-19: wait and hope." *Gyeonggi Multicultural Family News*, February 24, 2021. https://www.familynet.or.kr/download.do?uuid=abo88825-71a4-467b-b9eb-4c41607ac6bd.pdf.

Song, Heejin. 2013. "How international is EIL?: A critical discourse analysis of cultural representations in a Korean EFL education television program." *Critical Intersections in Education* 1, no. 2: 97–110.

Song, Juyoung. 2019. "*Wuli* and stance in a Korean heritage language classroom: A language socialization perspective." *Linguistics and Education* 51, no. 3: 12–19.

Suh, Kyung Hee, and Kyu-Hyun Kim. 2019. "Mitie tamhwauy piphancek tamhwapwunsek: tongnama icwumin kisalul cwungsimulo" [A critical discourse analysis of media discourse on Southeast Asian immigrants]. *Tamhwawa Inchi* 26, no. 3: 101–128.

World Health Organization. 2021. "Coronavirus disease (COVID-19) pandemic." https://www.who.int/emergencies/diseases/novel-coronavirus-2019.

Yoon, Jae Hak. 2003. "Tanswucek yongpepuy wuli" [The singular usage of *wuli*]. *Enewa Cengpo* 7, no. 2: 1–30.

CHAPTER 8

Movement Control Orders or "Making Confusing Orders"? Discourses of Confusion about Lockdowns in a Malaysian News Portal

Richard Powell & Zarina Othman

Abstract

Focusing on uses of the word "confusion" and its close cognates, this chapter adopts a Critical Discourse Analysis framework to examine stances behind references to COVID-19 lockdowns and other containment measures in reports and reader comments in the online news portal *Malaysiakini.* Although the language of confusion often conveys general feelings of disruption and disorientation in response to the health crisis and its administrative consequences, it also frequently encompasses criticism of the content, communication, or implementation of these measures, especially in opinion pieces or reader comments. While government policies inevitably attract censure in times of uncertainty, the authors argue that discourses of confusion are also employed to express frustration with a political crisis predating the health crisis itself.

Keywords: confusion, control orders, discourse analysis, health crisis, political critique

1. Motivation and Aims

As elsewhere, the lives of residents of Malaysia since early 2020 have been disrupted not only by the spread of COVID-19 itself but also by the regulations, restrictions and instructions which came with it. Malaysia's initial COVID-19 containment measures, gazetted in March 2020 as *Perintah Kawalan Pergerakan* (PKP) in Malay and the Movement Control Order (MCO) in English, closed non-essential businesses, restricted domestic movement, and suspended international travel. They also provided the basis for more targeted measures to deal with changing circumstances in different areas, including Continued Movement Control Orders (CMCOs) to prolong restrictions, Recovery Movement Control Orders (RMCOs) to ease them, and Enhanced Control Orders (EMCOs) to tighten them around high-infection clusters. The application of these measures to the complex details of everyday life has been a constant topic of media debate, much of it addressing the Standard Operating Procedures (SOPs) issued periodically to explain compliance.

In the second quarter of 2021, Malaysia began to slide down the Covid Resilience rankings as other countries rolled out enough vaccinations to control infections and ease restrictions (Hong, Chang, and Varley, 2021),[1] and while there were few anti-lockdown protests,[2] lockdowns have faced no shortage of criticism in the media. Some Malaysians view the control orders as repressive, others feel they do not go far enough, and many describe them as confusing.

Readers of the online news portal *Malaysiakini* have traded blackly humorous versions of the new acronyms, including Making Confusing Orders (MCOs), Continue Making Confusing Orders (CMCOs), Even More Confusing Orders (EMCOs) and Repeatedly Making Confusing Orders (RMCOs). The official Malay equivalents of these English acronyms, PKP (*Perintah Kawalan Pergerakan*), PKPB (*Perintah Kawalan Pergerakan Bersyarat*), PKPP (*Perintah Kawalan Pergerakan Pemulihan*) and PKPD (*Perintah Kawalan Pergerakan Diperketatkan*), were also subjected to lampooning.[3] *Sin Chew Daily* described regulations with a Chinese-Malay word 辛菜 [*cincai*] for "random" (Chong, 2021) and one local comedian, playing on the English acronym SOP and Malay word for soup (*sop*), used a cooking show format to parody VIPs getting away with violations which land ordinary citizens in the soup.[4] Using humour to make the best of a bad situation can be hazardous though, as when a Facebook user responded to a celebrity couple's getting away with an illegal cross-border trip with the wry comment: "I only just found out Nilai 3 is in Selangor" and the police investigated her for potentially causing "public alarm and confusion" (*Malaysiakini*, 2021e).

However much legal drafters strive for precise and autonomous texts, different interpretations are inevitable. There is perennial debate in legal philosophy about whether textual indeterminacy merely reflects the unavoidable vagueness of human language (Asgeirsson, 2015) or serves strategic purposes (Soames, 2012), such as allowing for flexible interpretation of laws in unpredictable circumstances (Endicott, 2011). Bhatia (1993) argues that if there is conflict between public accessibility and legal transparency the former is usually sacrificed, but emergency regulations need to prioritise public comprehension because of the potential consequences of non-compliance. This study explores the range of disruptive experiences indexed by public commentary on the confusing nature of regulations and their enforcement. While we will focus primarily on subjective responses—some linked to stances primed by cultural, social, or political events going beyond the regulations themselves—there may be pointers for drafters attempting to make rules more intelligible objectively. The discourses of confusion in our data suggest that this task is particularly challenging if the recipients of instructions view authorities as untrustworthy or incompetent.

2. Background to the MCOs

Malaysia's first Movement Control Order (later dubbed MCO 1.0) was announced on television in March 2020 by Prime Minister Muhyiddin Yassin and widely translated into English, Chinese, and other languages. Schools, places of worship and non-essential retailers were to be closed (*New Straits Times*, 2020a) and entry into or exit from the country prohibited. The legal framing of the Order included the Police Act, 1967 and the Prevention and Control of Infectious Diseases Act, 1988, the latter allowing for fines of 1000 ringgit (about US$250) for violations. On the eve of implementation there were reports of public confusion as university students flooded bus terminals, unsure of whether they required a permit to return to their hometowns (Bernama.com, 2020). On March 25, the Prime Minister announced the first of a series of extensions, and on the same day an Enhanced Movement Control Order (EMCO) imposed home confinement in areas of high infection (Astrowani. com, 2020). On March 30 the Senior Minister for the Security Cluster lengthened the operating hours for essential businesses (*Borneo Post*, 2020) and on April 10 this category was extended to hardware and electrical stores (*New Straits Times*, 2020b). Following the announcement of a Continued Movement Control Order (CMCO) on May 1, the coming weeks saw a number of modifications to the original Order to allow greater economic activity within publicly announced Standard Operating Procedures (SOPs) for social distancing, and the use of tracking apps. A petition against the CMCO garnered 429,000 signatures (*Malay Mail*, 2020).

With signs of improved conditions, a Recovery Movement Control Order (RMCO) announced in June (*New Straits Times Online*, 2020) allowed interstate domestic travel, swimming, and outdoor food sales (Loo, 2020) and in July, family entertainment facilities were reopened (Mazwin, 2020). The following month the RMCO was extended until the end of the year (*New Straits Times*, 2020c), but in November a tighter CMCO was reinstated for the capital and several other states, including Sabah, where state elections had been held in September despite the risk of crowd-spread infections (Latiff, 2020). In the same month, attempts were made to set up travel bubbles in states where infections were lower (Vincent Tan, 2020).

With cases on the rise again, the RMCO was extended until the end of March (*Channel News Asia*, 2021), with a more comprehensive MCO (MCO 2.0) imposed in western Malaya and Sabah (Nadirah, 2021) that banned interstate travel and intrastate trips over ten kilometres from home, limited restaurants to takeaway service and restricted religious gatherings. A State of Emergency declared on the same day (*Ordinan Darurat Kuasa-Kuasa Perlu*) suspended parliament and extended the government's executive powers (PMO, 2020). Since independence in 1957, seven emergency ordinances have been imposed, most to contain political disorder, and this one attracted speculation as to whether it was primarily a political move to shore up a minority government (Loh, 2021) rather than a health measure (*Bernama/Malaysiakini*, 2021a), given that Malaysian politics had been particularly volatile in the preceding years.

While holding regular elections since independence, for sixty years the nation was ruled continuously by a coalition dominated by the United Malays National Organisation (UMNO), with opposition parties held in check largely by government domination of patronage and state media. In 2018, voters ended this continuity amidst a massive high-ranking corruption scandal, and the ensuing political disruption lingers. The incoming Pakatan Harapan government, an alliance between opposition parties and UMNO renegades, collapsed within two years (Razak and Zakiah, 2020) under a wave of defections. Its successor, the Perikatan Nasional minority coalition, comprising several religious and regional parties alongside defectors from Pakatan Harapan, emerged from backroom negotiations on the eve of the pandemic in February 2020 and its legitimacy remained questionable until it too was replaced by another minority coalition in August 2021. Elections in November 2022 have since brought Pakatan back into power in an unlikely coalition with a weakened UMNO.

Already riding ongoing political tensions, Perikatan Nasional raised the temperature of political debate about the impartiality and clarity of SOP enforcement when it amended the State of Emergency Ordinance so as to increase fines for violators to 10,000 ringgit (US $2,500) (*The Star*, 2021). In another hotly debated amendment on March 11 the government curbed the spread of what it considered fake news, overriding the Evidence Act, 1950 and reinstating many of the measures in an anti-fake-news act which had been repealed by their predecessors (*Malaysiakini*, 2021b). Two months later, after several weeks of easing, another comprehensive control order, MCO 3.0, was imposed nationwide (*Malaysiakini*, 2021c), since rebranded as the National Recovery Plan.

3. Data Collection and Analysis

Malaysiakini was chosen as the main data source partly because of the above average levels of trust and large number of digital readers it enjoys domestically (Reuters Institute, 2019), and partly because of its positive international reputation (Yang and Leong, 2016). Additional background information about the control orders has been taken from other Malaysian as well as international news sources. Malaysia as a whole ranks poorly for press freedom (Reporters without Borders, 2021), which may help explain why *Malaysiakini* is frequently criticised by the government. Reader comments on the portal are relatively unreserved and in February 2021 led to the portal being convicted for contempt of court (Lim, 2021).

This study emerged from perusal of the portal's English edition, which generally explains any Malay terms appearing in news stories but leaves Malay and code-mixes intact in reader comments. Described officially as "a strong second language" (Government of Malaysia, 1976, p. 384), English is taught as a subject in nearly all schools and widely used as a medium at secondary and tertiary level as well as in many non-governmental domains, but one comment in the data recommended greater use of Malay to explain technical information (*Malaysiakini*, 2021a).

The authentic versions of MCOs, as with all post-1967 legislation, are in Malay, with official 'translations' in English, although there is evidence that the practice of drafting in English first and then translating into Malay remains common (Powell, 2020). Our inquiry began by using *Malaysiakini*'s keyword search function for "confuse," and the variants "confuses," "confused," "confusing," and "confusion" in articles related to movement restrictions for the year following the announcement of the first MCO on March 16, 2020. This produced sixty-six relevant articles, half of them news reports and the others commentaries contributed by politicians, journalists, or readers, the total corpus amounting to some 41,500 words. We included readers' comments on articles if they contained "confuse" or any of its variants. Extending the data by two months would have encompassed a surge of reporting and commentary on the third nationwide Movement Control Order, but by March the target lexeme had already produced a large enough range of co-texts and contexts, so we also excluded articles using semiotically similar terms (such as "misleading," "unclear," or "vague"), or code-mixed Malay terms (such as *pusing-pusing*). For background information, however, we do refer to some reports falling outside the twelve-month period. We also looked at the Malay-language pages of *Malaysiakini* over the same period for the contexts of *keliru* (confuse) and *kekeliruan* (confusion) in MCO-related stories to gauge whether they were being used in similar ways.

Instances of "confuse" and variants were analysed for the surrounding topic and also for the stance of the speech acts in which they were embedded. Articles analysed in the corpus are listed separately, after the list of references.

4. Findings

4.1. Text Genres

Half (33) of the articles were presented as news reports, some with named bylines. Many of these carried statements from government ministers announcing or defending MCO-related polices juxtaposed with critical comments from politicians (generally from opposition parties) or representatives of business, health, educational, or cultural bodies. Nine of them were uncritical explanations of movement control measures and Standard Operating Procedures.

Many of the articles had "confuse" or a variant in the headline itself, such as explanatory pieces accompanying the announcement of new orders (e.g., "Confused? Here's where and when to wear facemasks," *Malaysiakini*, 2020h) and including visuals to clarify rules. Others reported on social confusion or allegations of confusion.

Eleven articles were commentaries penned by politicians, political analysts, academics, or figures from business, education, or science, and carried disclaimers that the views were independent of the portal. Several more were round-ups of readers' comments on specific MCO-related topics. These appeared more frequently following the issuance of a new Order or during controversy over related Standard Operating Procedures. Where there were readers' comments there might be entire threads on confusion about new rules or their enforcement.

5. Recurring Topics

5.1 Travel Restrictions

The most common topic attracting the language of confusion was travel. On the eve of the first MCO, students were reported trying to return to their hometowns before the capital was locked down and crowding bus stations, unsure whether they needed police permits. One opposition politician's description of "confusing instructions as well as u-turns" (*Malaysiakini*, 2020a) and another's demand for "complete and not confusing information" (*Malayskiakini*, 2020b) preceded readers' comments on rules which were "confusing and not properly detailed out" (*Malaysiakini*, 2020c). The Malay version of this story (Aw, 2020) describes the instructions to students as *tidak jelas* (not clear) but also adds a statement from the Higher Education Minister in which she describes her failure to comment on National Security Council orders as an attempt to avoid adding to the confusion.

The SOP regulating state border crossings soon emerged as a hot topic. Many Malaysians who had rushed back to their hometowns when travel restrictions were first announced found themselves stranded from their workplaces, and in April the Malay edition of *Malaysiakini* carried the Security Cluster Minister's comments about the public themselves causing confusion (*Bernama/Malaysiakini*, 2020a). Under MCO 2.0, which ushered in heavier penalties, the Defence Minister was reported to be "ironing out a confusion" over the crossing of district borders which appeared differently on state and police maps (*Malaysiakini*, 2021s), while readers made much of confusing boundaries and confused implementation (*Malaysiakini*, 2021t).

Also contentious were limits on passengers in private vehicles. Framed in one article as evidence of flexibility, the possibility that "two people" might mean two per vehicle for multi-car households, or that babies did not count, was described in reader comments as confusing and open to subjective enforcement (*Malaysiakini*, 2020l). Several articles dealt with the regulation of travel to workplaces by work sector. "Mass confusion" was reported when police stopped issuing travel permits after the government waived this requirement for those in possession of an employer's letter, apparently without informing relevant parties about the change (Ramieza Wahid, 2020). In October, an opposition politician condemned a work-from-home directive as "too general and confusing" and bringing economic hardship (*Malaysiakini*, 2020i), and the portal put out a detailed explanation of procedures such as swab tests after commenting that there had been "a lot of confusion" (*Malaysiakini*, 2020i). An advisor to the government's own sovereign wealth fund also characterised work-from-home orders as confusing (Tong, 2020).

5.2 Work Management

In the early days of the first MCO, the Federation of Malaysian Freight Forwarders demanded clarity about whether its work was considered essential and what medical and administrative procedures were required to get through police roadblocks (*Malaysiakini*, 2020e). Confusion over the need for drivers to use a government-authorised tracing app before refuelling was reported after a minister said it was "required in some circumstances but not in others" (*Malaysiakini*, 2020m). Access to private condominiums also became a source of confusion after managers and security guards were reported having difficulty interpreting the SOPs regarding the entry of realtors and prospective or even newly confirmed tenants (Low, 2021).

At the beginning of 2021, long-standing confusion about work-from-home instructions was related in a letter in the portal's Malay pages, with *runsing* (puzzled), *bertukar-tukar* (changing) and *bimbang* (concerned) contextually linked with *keliru* (*Malaysiakini*, 2021v). The letter condemned the inconsistency of imposing a work-from-home regime in October and one week later allowing sports centres to open without granting exemption permits to employees.

5.3 Social Distancing and Mask Wearing

During MCO 1.0 an academic described the difficulty authorities worldwide had in agreeing on appropriate distances (Low. 2021). A government minister commented on confusion amongst the public and restaurateurs regarding table spacing (*Bernama/Malaysiakini* 2020b). Slow investigations of apparent violations of SOPs by politicians and other well-known figures sharing meals at close proximity triggered lively commentary from readers, many confessing sardonically to confusion about inconsistent enforcement (*Malaysiakini*, 2021f, 2021r; *Bernama/Malaysiakini*, 2021b). One story carrying questions from a disgraced former prime minister about the legality of a birthday celebration for an opposition politician was met with a reader's comments about the "chaos and confusion" of the SOPs (Low, 2021).

Mask wearing was a further source of claims of confusion. In a letter published after masks were made mandatory in public, an opposition politician claimed "even enforcement officers are confused" (Lee, 2020), echoing readers' comments about the police being confused after a teenager was fined for pulling down his mask while waiting for a train (Lee, 2020). Following a notorious case in which condominium managers fined an unmasked one-year-old, a government minister clarified that only the police and the Ministry of Health were authorised to issue fines, but he was rebuffed by one reader for confusing the public and by another for frequently changing regulations (Faisal Asyraf, 2021). Allegations of skewed enforcement surged in the wake of the increased fines which followed the declaration of a State of Emergency, particularly when the government offered a reduction for first-time offenders without clarifying how to claim it (*Malaysiakini*, 2021u). This situation prompted one reader to comment that confusion could have been avoided if the regime for fines had been included in the original ordinance rather than provided for ex post facto (Alyaa Alhadjri, 2021).

5.4 Medical Information

Confusion was frequently mentioned in connection with medical matters. One story described suspected COVID-19 sufferers unable to get advice from the Ministry of Health on how to prepare for hospitalisation (Lee and Hariz, 2020). Another targeted public misconception about the spread of infection and the need for greater clarity about the safe discharge of recovered patients (Ramieza Wahid, 2021a). A third story covered government threats to fine clinics for late reporting of test results, with the president of the Malaysian Medical Association blaming the Health Department's confusing SOPs for the delays (*Malaysiakini*, 2021j). The media was also accused of creating confusion when the National Disaster Management Agency objected to interpretations of images of an apparently chaotic quarantine centre (*Malaysiakini*, 2021g). Prior to the vaccination programme the portal reported a leading medic's call for the government and relevant NGOs to dispel the confusion caused by anti-vaccine advocates (*Bernama/Malaysiakini*, 2020c), and a more general article sought to shed light on confusing comparisons of different vaccines (*Reuters/Malaysiakini*, 2020). With the State of Emergency, warnings against politicising health management also began to appear, one commentator describing it as "not a help but a hindrance because it adds further uncertainty to an already confusing situation" (Oh, 2021).

5.5 Cultural Practices and Social Activities

The SOPs for travel to and gatherings at cultural and religious events often drew claims of confusion. Discussion about who could visit whom, where, and in the company of how many escalated in the run up to Chinese New Year (*Malaysiakini*, 2021l; 2021m; 2021n), with one opposition spokesman warning that a lack of a clear policy for all communities could court allegations of favouring politics over health (Ramieza Wahid, 2021b). One commenter compared restrictions on the Chinese community with earlier tolerance for night markets (*Malaysiakini*, 2021l), which many readers might take to refer to Malay gatherings during Ramadhan.

Other topics framed within discourses of confusion included provisions for the holding of school exams (*Malaysiakini*, 2021o; M Fakrul Halim, 2021) and for NGO and volunteer activities (Nathaniel Tan, 2020). There were also sporadic reports on administrative or economic matters which indirectly referred to the challenges posed by control orders. For example, a report on confusion amongst agents involved with arranging residence visas for foreigners was contextualised by a reminder of how the programme had been disrupted with the suspension of entry from abroad under MCO 1.0 (*Malaysiakini*, 2020g).

5.6 Dissemination of Information

Not long into MCO 1.0 the control of information took centre stage in the battle against the pandemic, with the government threatening to reinstate anti-fake-news legislation and human rights groups calling its definition of fake news "unclear and confusing" (Alyaa Alhadjiri, 2020). Civil society groups concerned about freedom of expression called the government's definition of fake "unclear and confusing" (*Malaysiakini*, 2020f). The portal also published more widely framed articles on the role of information. One columnist questioned the medical and psychological value of the term "social distancing," given the need for physical distance but social solidarity at "this confusing and challenging time" (Surin, 2020). An academic devoted an article to "misinformation, disinformation and rumours during a health emergency [which] can hamper public health responses by creating confusion and distrust" (Mohammad Firdaus, 2020). An opposition politician accused authorities of making people confused through "unnecessary announcements" (*Malaysiakini*, 2020k), and after ridiculing inconsistent SOPs as *Semua Orang Pening* (everyone is dizzy), a former Finance Minister described them as making a dire situation even more confusing (*Malaysiakini*, 2021q). One reader summarised the difficulties people had about SOPs with: "Too many ifs and buts. Too many lines. Confusing. Keep it Simple." (*Malaysiakini*, 2021i).

In defence of his government, one minister dismissed public confusion as the result of impatience with instructions explicitly stated to be provisional (*Malaysiakini*, 2020j). An Australian academic, while acknowledging the confusion many Malaysians felt over apparent conflicts between federal measures and local state provisions, pointed out that individual states enjoyed an autonomy which enabled them to respond appropriately to local situations (Welsh, 2020).

5.7 Communicative Function and Stance

Moving from contexts to co-texts, and from topics to illocution, the data highlight the range of communicative functions which discourses of confusion may serve. Thirty-eight functioned as speech acts which could be considered complaints; eleven invoked demands, with another nuanced as a request. There were three instances of warning against confusion and three of advising about how to overcome it, as well as three cases praising measures or communications which avoided confusion. There were also twenty-eight speech acts in which confusion was reported without any discernible stance.

While it is difficult to gauge stance in complex interdiscursive texts such as news articles, with their selective reporting and journalistic distancing strategies, just over half of the English articles appeared broadly critical of government policy or practice, while a further four appraised police enforcement negatively. Criticism of the government also featured prominently in Malay articles, many of them embracing sarcasm to admonish authorities. In defending itself, the government also referred to confusion: *Ada kekeliruan ... yang ada di bandar nak balik ke kampung tidak boleh, daripada awal lagi kita beritahu tidak boleh* (There was confusion...those staying in the cities are not allowed to go back to their hometowns, we informed them of this from the beginning) (*Bernama/Malaysiakini*, 2020a). One article singled out business interests for blame and another chastised the media. Four articles revolved around criticisms voiced by government representatives, two of these targeting public conduct in general, one warning against rumour-mongering, and the fourth chiding condominium managers. Confusion was also indexed in two expressions of support for authorities, with some articles praising the police in view of the confusing nature of the orders they had to carry out (Yi, 2020).

In contrast, readers' allegations of confusion were rarely linked to positive appraisals of the authorities. Many, cast as confessions of personal disorientation, were clearly intended to criticise the duplicity of people in positions of authority. Against this general negativity, the Director-General of Health was sometimes singled out for avoiding the confusion associated with other government figures (Bhatia, 2020). Despite the title *Buat SOP biarlah masuk akal* (Be logical when constructing SOP) (Ibrahim Ali, 2020), one Malay letter was generally positive about the Ministry of Health's initiatives, reserving its comments about confusion for frequent changes in the SOPs accompanying them.

The minority of texts which indexed confusion without ascribing human agency were either explanatory pieces to clarify regulations, or somewhat-personal accounts of the socioeconomic disruption and psychological disorientation the pandemic induced. One contribution about the importance of maintaining mental health, for example, acknowledged how confusing it was to follow multiple regulations, while nonetheless emphasising the necessity of doing so (Aziz Ahmad, 2020). Another described the confused feelings of people experiencing economic dislocation (Fa Abdul, 2020). A senior police officer conceded that some measures might have been enforced inconsistently, but put this down to human propensity to interpret complex rules in different ways, especially when they embodied sufficient flexibility to respond to changing circumstances (*Malaysiakini*, 2021p). In a more specific vein, readers' discussion about the timing of new rules included the comment "Many confused midnight as the start of a new date, others the end of that date," and although another recommended imitating the airlines in choosing times like 11:59 p.m. or 12:01 a.m., no authority was singled out for blame (*Malaysiakini*, 2021h).

5.8 Confusion as Political Critique

The chief human targets of claims of confusion were the government departments formulating policy, the government spokesmen issuing and explaining policy, and the police and other authorities enforcing it. While *Malaysiakini* reported Prime Minister Muhyiddin's announcement of the first MCO as "well-received" on social media, it contrasted this with an account of the chaos which ensued as citizens struggled to understand practical details (*Malaysiakini*, 2020a). Reader comments could be particularly censorious of inconsistent messages, such as when one official told people to scan into a tracing app before buying petrol, a senior police officer said this was unnecessary when paying through a window, and a government minister added that it depended on whether the queue was "long" (*Malaysiakini*, 2020l). Many criticisms targeted the wording of MCOs and SOPs themselves, with one opinion article calling for "much more clarity about the never-ending stream of extremely confusing—and thus extremely frustrating—movement control order (MCO) policies" (Nathaniel Tan, 2020).

With the government bearing the brunt of criticism, we often find confusion functioning as a trope for political critique which questions the underlying competency and even legitimacy of the government. There are parallels here with the employment of "confusion" to delegitimise ideological opponents discussed by Khan and Samuel (2020) in their analysis of op-eds about faith-based conflict in Malaysia. While they find confusion weaponised in religious and communal debate, in our data it was linked to the installation of an unstable and controversial minority government (Tan and Azmi, 2021).

The potential for politicised use of confusion appeared early on in the pandemic when a former deputy prime minister called on authorities to issue "complete and not confusing information" to lessen panic (*Malaysiakini* 2020a). Ostensibly pragmatic in taking up the confusion of students crowding bus stations, his demand that the government be "more responsible and ethical" was arguably an attempt to link incomplete instructions to deeper political turmoil. Similarly, in an article condemning official "announcements and pronouncements that, if not utterly confusing or meant to confuse, would surely have obfuscated the situation" (Bhatia, 2020), a research scholar described the government as an "interloper," a reference to its controversial formation. One critic implied that ad hoc and reactive pandemic measures were not only a sign of incompetence but also a strategy to control the public (Raj, 2020). Some opposition politicians were also associated negatively with confusion. In response to a parliamentarian's complaint that the government was imposing heavier penalties on ordinary citizens for violations of vague regulations which senior figures were themselves circumventing, one reader commented: "Opposition will talk exact opposite to government actions. Confuse the people. Enough of political talk" (*Malaysiakini*, 2021k).

6. Discussion

Although many claims of confusion in the corpus encompassed neutral or self-reflective accounts devoid of agency, most incorporated a critical stance towards people, institutions, or human practices. Describing stance as "undeniably complex," Du Bois (2007, p. 173) emphasises its diachronic and dialogic dimensions, and Khan and Samuel (2020) refer to a history of ideologised assertions of confusion in Malaysia designed to delegitimise other worldviews and accuse opponents of deliberate obfuscation. In this study we tried not to stray far from the immediate context of control orders, but the stance of many reports and comments can be linked to the wider context of political confusion.

The unnamed editorial pieces tended to assume a neutral stance which cast confusion as understandable yet mitigable, such as an explanation of mask wearing (*Malaysiakini*, 2020h) which includes the word "confused?" in the headline to establish a rapport with readers.

Editorials further differed from news reports in addressing readers directly. In a corpus split fairly evenly between reports and commentaries, it may be significant that it was news articles which contained twenty-two of the thirty tokens of "confusion" (rather than "confused" or "confusing"), suggesting that nominalisation aids distancing. News reports are highly intertextual, however, invariably containing direct or indirect quotations, and many of the reports in this data encompassed more subtle positioning in their selection of cited informants. Even though government ministers are given space to blame others for confusion in the corpus, an underlying antipathy to the government is apparent, and in addition to the selection of comments, *Malaysiakini*'s news reports themselves construct stances lexicogrammatically: "Dazed and confused: Covid-19 positive patients wait at home in limbo" (Lee and Hariz, 2020).

Over a third of the texts are by invited contributors, five of them from the world of media, communications, or policy analysis, four from politics (all in the opposition), three from academia, and two from other professions. This range of backgrounds is reflected in a range of stances, with politicians characteristically attacking government policies or policy enforcement, adopting the moral high ground and accusing the government of issuing "confusing instructions" (*Malaysiakini*, 2020a) which leave law enforcers themselves "confused" (Lee, 2020). As might be expected, the commentaries of academics are less politicised and tend to frame criticism of policies within more abstract language and a broader perspective.

Readers' comments, which appear largely to be unedited, are mostly informal, and some are code-mixed ("Police are confused, Rakyat [public] are confused but Summons *tetap jalan* [keep coming]" (*Malaysiakini*, 2021k)). Sarcasm is rife, and even when personal confusion is admitted, the admission may be barbed: "Please enlighten this confused citizen... many thanks" (*Malaysiakini*, 2021r). Interdiscursivity is more transparent in the comments than in the other text genres as readers engage directly not only with the content of an article but also with other readers.

While undoubtedly a tool of complaint and criticism, the attribution of confusion to policies, policy communication, and policy enforcement also reflects the complexity of life under a pandemic and the weaknesses, whether intellectual or moral, of individuals. It consequently offers pointers for how confusion might be reduced by revising policies and practices. Many contributor and reader comments embrace the possibility of improvement by evaluating some officials or offices more favourably than others or comparing Malaysian and foreign practices. Yet authorities may have a hard time drawing lessons from the ideologised labelling of policy-makers themselves as confused.

7. Conclusions

The COVID-19 pandemic brought disruption to daily life on a scale rarely experienced outside wartime, and it is hardly surprising that claims of confusion were widespread. When we look at the *Malaysiakini* data we see the term used to describe a wide range of dislocations in readers' sense of health and safety, socioeconomic security, and civic loyalty. We also see it used as a call for disruption in response to regulations and practices which are perceived either as ill-wrought or enforced in bad faith.

The diversity apparent in these discourses of confusion highlights the importance of socio-political contexts for policy-makers when aiming to maximise compliance. This study suggests that the more concrete conceptualisations of confusion offer lessons for improving policy and policy reception, even though they figure prominently amongst the more critical commentary in the data. When health-related worries and socioeconomic disruption are entangled with personalised, disembodied, or ideologised stances, however, it may be particularly difficult for regulatory bodies to increase the clarity of their instructions.

The perennial need of authorities to mitigate the ambiguity of legislation has a particular urgency to it in the context of emergency regulations. In addition to the legal transparency and impartiality required of any enactment, such measures need to be accessible to the general public without the mediation of legal experts. The aphorism about ignorance being no defence in law may have legal validity, but its socio-political validity is limited if confusion puts the health of society at risk. The avoidance of confusion calls for keeping things simple. But textual simplicity and interpretative clarity are not always the same thing, and legal readability may run along a different trajectory from general readability. Drafting measures to deal with rapidly changing situations also calls for flexibility, but this may in turn open the door to uncertainty. In short, the task of generating effective control measures during crises is fraught with difficulty, and it is hardly surprising that confusion features prominently in the discourse.

Malaysian authorities, like those elsewhere, have had at least three battles to fight under this pandemic: containing the virus; sustaining the economy; and maintaining public trust and cooperation. And as movement restrictions continue, economic malaise deepens, and death tolls rise, success in the first two may become increasingly dependent on success in the third. Towards the end of his term of office, Perikatan Nasional Prime Minister Muhyiddin highlighted the crucial role of voluntary collaboration, emphasising that there are not enough enforcement officers to ensure all 30 million Malaysians abide by regulations and eliminate all suspicion of double standards (*Malaysiakini*, 2021d). However, the persuasiveness of the message may have been attenuated by additional comments he made about confusion arising from "the changing nature of the Covid-19 virus," which may have been factually relevant but risked being interpreted as avoidance of responsibility.

After reviewing Lawrence Wright's *The Plague Year*, Sonali Deraniyagala concludes "Our response to catastrophe is often bewilderment ... While our personal confusion about these unimaginable events will always linger, we are grateful for the clarity that comes from trying to comprehend the larger story" (Deraniyagala, 2021). This is unlikely to be the last pandemic in our lifetimes. It remains to be seen whether it will turn out to be the most confusing.

Richard Powell, Professor at Nihon University and Vice-President of the Japan Association of Law and Language, researches forensic linguistics, legal English, language planning and cross-cultural pragmatics in East Africa and East, South and Southeast Asia, recently authoring *Language Choice in Postcolonial Law: Lessons from Malaysia's Bilingual Legal System* (Springer, 2020).

Zarina Othman is Associate Professor at Universiti Kebangsaan, Malaysia. Dr. Zarina's research interests include the study of academic discourse, linguistics sexism, ELT and ESP Teaching, and Language and Communication. She is currently the Secretary to MAAL, the Malaysian Association of Applied Linguistics.

Notes

1 Number 20 on Bloomberg's Covid Resilience Ranking of 53 on April 26; as of June 29 it was ranked at 51, overtaken by countries that have managed to control infection levels while also easing movement restrictions.
2 Some *Malaysiakini* readers have suggested the lockdown controls themselves, rather than the willingness to comply with them, explain the lack of street protests, with the police dealing harshly in July 2021 with protesters calling for the resignation of the Prime Minister amidst growing infections.
3 For example, a scene from the iconic 1964 film Madu Tiga was circulated on social media after being redubbed to have the main characters discuss the complexities of the different control orders.
4 "DUDUK TV with CHEF WANTU BAKEMAISHU" https://www.youtube.com/watch?v=PBCz248B3U4.

References

Asgeirsson, Hrafn. 2015. "On the instrumental value of vagueness in the law." *Ethics* 125, no. 2: 425–448.

Astrowani.com. 2020. "COVID-19: PKPD dikuat kuasa di dua kawasan di Simpang Renggam" [COVID-19: EMCO enforced in two areas in Simpang Renggam]. March 26, 2020. https://www.astroawani.com/berita-malaysia/covid19-pkpd-dikuat-kuasa-di-dua-kawasan-di-simpang-renggam-235454.

Bernama.com. 2020. "COVID-19: Public to inform police for interstates travel." March 17, 2020. https://www.bernama.com/en/news.php?id=1822162.

Bernama/Malaysiakini. 2021a. "Parliament postponed on legal grounds to aid fight against Covid-19 – Takiyuddin." March 3, 2021. https://www.malaysiakini.com/news/565158.

Bhatia, Vijay. 1993. *Analysing Genre: Language Use in Professional Settings*. London/New York: Longman.

Borneo Post. 2020. "New business hours 8am-8pm for premises selling essential items starting April 1 – Ismail Sabri." March 30, 2020. https://www.theborneopost.com/2020/03/30/mco-new-business-hours-8am-8pm-for-premises-selling-essential-items-starting-april-1-ismail-sabri/.

Channel News Asia. 2021. "COVID-19: Malaysia's recovery movement control order extended again to Mar 31." January 21, 2021. https://www.channelnewsasia.com/news/asia/malaysia-covid-19-rmco-extended-mar-31-restrictions-13877484.

Chong, Lip Teck. 2021. MCO: Malaysia Cincai Order. Sinchew News.com, 10 May 2021. https://www.sinchew.com.my/content/content_2474989.html.

Deraniyagala, Sonali. 2021. "Review of The Plague Year." *New York Times*, June 7, 2021. https://www.nytimes.com/2021/06/07/books/review/lawrence-wright-the-plague-year.html.

Du Bois, John. 2007. "The stance triangle." In *Stancetaking in Discourse: Subjectivity, Evaluation, Interaction*, edited by Robert Englebretson, 139–182. John Benjamins.

Endicott, Timothy. 2011. "Vagueness and law." In *Vagueness: A Guide*, edited by Giuseppina Ronzitti, 171–191. Logic, Epistemology and the Unit of Science 19.

Government of Malaysia. 1976. *Third Malaysia Plan, 1976-80*. https://policy.asiapacificenergy.org/sites/default/files/3rd%20MP.pdf.

Hong, Jinshan, Rachel Chang, and Kevin Varley. 2021. *The Covid Resilience Ranking: The Best and Worst Places to Be as Variants Outrace Vaccinations*. https://www.bloomberg.com/graphics/covid-resilience-ranking/.

Khan, Mahmud Hasan, and Moses Stephens Gunams Samuel. 2020. "Confusion as an ideological tool in Malaysian newspaper op-eds." *CROSSINGS 11*: 225–241.

Latiff, Rozanna. 2020. "Malaysian leaders draw flak after post-election virus jump. " Reuters, October 2, 2020. https://www.reuters.com/article/us-health-coronavirus-malaysia/malaysian-leaders-draw-flak-after-post-election-virus-jump-idUSKBN26N1SP.

Lim, Ida. 2021. "In Malaysiakini decision, Federal Court acknowledges spotlight on free speech but reminds Malaysians to be polite online." *The Malay Mail*, February 19, 2021. https://www.malaymail.com/news/malaysia/2021/02/19/in-malaysiakini-decision-federal-court-acknowledges-spotlight-on-free-speec/1951082.

Loh, Jason. 2021. "Is the state of emergency justifiable at the end of the day?" *The Malay Mail*, January 15, 2021. https://www.malaymail.com/news/what-you-think/2021/01/15/is-the-state-of-emergency-justifiable-at-the-end-of-the-day-jason-loh/1940618.

Loo, Cindi. 2020. "CMCO ends June 9. Recovery MCO from June 10 to Aug 31." *The Sun Daily*, June 7, 2020. https://www.thesundaily.my/home/cmco-ends-june-9-recovery-mco-from-june-10-to-aug-31-updated-EM2538754

Malay Mail. 2020. "Over 420,000 Malaysians sign petition objecting to CMCO which starts tomorrow." May 3, 2020. https://www.malaymail.com/news/malaysia/2020/05/03/over-420000-malaysians-sign-petition-objecting-to-cmco-which-starts-tomorro/1862546.

Malaysiakini. 2021a. "Singapore suspends travel bubble with Malaysia." January 30, 2021. https://www.malaysiakini.com/news/560996.

Malaysiakini. 2021b. "Emergency Ordinance grants Putrajaya sweeping powers against 'fake news.'" March 11, 2021. https://www.malaysiakini.com/news/566220.

Malaysiakini. 2021c. "It's back to nationwide MCO from May 12." May 10, 2021. https://www.malaysiakini.com/news/574152.

Malaysiakini. 2021d. "PM on SOP breach: Some got away due to lack of enforcers, but no double standards." May 23, 2021. https://www.malaysiakini.com/news/575848.

Malaysiakini. 2021e. "Nilai 3 is in S'gor' joke fails to tickle police's funny bone, probe initiated." May 24, 2021. https://www.malaysiakini.com/news/575864.

Malaysiakini. 2021f. "Rashid admits to attending durian feast recently, not last year." June 30, 2021. https://www.malaysiakini.com/news/581105.

Mazwin Nil Anis. 2020. "Family entertainment centres can reopen from July 15, says Ismail Sabri." *The Star*, July 10, 2020. https://www.thestar.com.my/news/nation/2020/07/10.

Nadirah H. Rodzi. 2021. "Malaysia to impose MCO for two weeks in several states to curb Covid-19 cases – Muhyiddin." *The Straits Times*, January 11, 2021. https://www.straitstimes.com/asia/se-asia/malaysia-to-impose-mco-for-2-weeks-from-jan-13-in-several-states-to-curb-covid-19-cases.

New Straits Times. 2020a. "Covid-19: Movement Control Order imposed with only essential sectors operating." March 16, 2020.

New Straits Times. 2020b. "Certain businesses given green light to operate during MCO." April 10, 2020.

New Straits Times. 2020c. "NST Leader: RMCO extension the right move." August 29, 2020.

New Straits Times Online. 2020. "[LIVE] Special address by Prime Minister on the Recovery Movement Control Order (RMCO)." YouTube video. June 7, 2020. https://www.youtube.com/watch?v=btE-fafQobeg.

PMO. 2020. Office of Prime Minister of Malaysia. Special Announcement of Emergency. https://www.pmo.gov.my/2021/01/teks-ucapan-pengumuman-khas-darurat/.

Powell, Richard. 2020. *Language Choice in Postcolonial Law: Lessons from Malaysia's Bilingual System*. Singapore: Springer.

Razak Ahmad, and Zakiah Koya. 2020. "Pakatan Harapan govt collapses." *The Star*, February 24, 2020. https://www.thestar.com.my/news/nation/2020/02/24/pakatan-harapan-govt-collapses.

Reporters without Borders. 2021. *World Press Freedom Index*. https://rsf.org/en/ranking/2021.

Reuters Institute. 2019. *Digital News Report* 2019, 138-139. https://reutersinstitute.politics.ox.ac.uk/sites/default/files/inline-files/DNR_2019_FINAL.pdf.

Soames, Scott. 2012. "Vagueness and the law." In *The Routledge Companion to Philosophy of Law*, edited by Andrei Marmor, 95–108. New York: Routledge, 2012.

Tan, Vincent. 2020. "Domestic travel bubbles approved in Malaysia as movement curbs lifted in four states." *Channel New Asia*, November 20, 2020. https://www.channelnewsasia.com/news/asia/malaysia-covid-19-domestic-travel-bubble-ismail-sabri-cmco-13601880.

The Star. 2021. "MCO violators face up to RM10,000 fine under amended Emergency Ordinance from March 11." February 25, 2021. https://www.thestar.com.my/news/nation/2021/02/25/rm10000-fine-for-mco-offences-under-new-emergency-ordinance-from-march-21.

Yang Lai Fong, and Wai Kit Leong. 2016. "Different political beliefs and different frame building for an inter-religious conflict: A comparative analysis of The Star and Malaysiakini." *Global Media Journal*, 2016. https://www.globalmediajournal.com/open-access/different-political-beliefs-and-d.

Texts Analysed in the Corpus

Alyaa Alhadjri. 2020. "Groups say gov't's fake news awareness alert 'unclear, confusing.'" *Malaysiakini*, April 11, 2020. https://www.malaysiakini.com/news/520068.

Alyaa Alhadjri. 2021. "Bukit Mertajam MP claims no guidelines to appeal RM10k fine." *Malaysiakini*, March 14, 2021. https://www.malaysiakini.com/news/566552.

Aw, Nigel. 2020. "Padah tersilap langkah, jangkitan Covid-19 berisiko melambung [Wrong move, Covid-19 infection at risk of soaring]. " *Malaysiakini*, March 18, 2020. https://www.malaysiakini.com/news/515266.

Aziz Ahmad. 2020. "Letter: Tired and exhausted at home." *Malaysiakini*, April 3, 2020. https://www.malaysiakini.com/letters/518567.

Bernama/Malaysiakini. 2020a. "Permohonan rentas negeri hanya untuk warga kandas di kampung [Cross-state applications only for residents stranded in their hometowns]." April 23, 2020. https://www.malaysiakini.com/news/522199.

Bernama/Malaysiakini. 2020b. "Recovery MCO: Take stern action against nightclubs, pubs – Ismail Sabri." September 14, 2020. https://www.malaysiakini.com/news/542619.

Bernama/Malaysiakini. 2020c. "Covid-19 vaccine safety: Transparency vital to avoid public confusion", December 1, 2020. https://www.malaysiakini.com/news/553282.

Bernama/Malaysiakini. 2021b. "Annuar's SOP violation case: Police to record statements from witnesses." February 18, 2021. https://www.malaysiakini.com/news/563393.

Bhatia, Manjit. 2020. "A voice of reason and reassurance in Covid-19 fight." *Malaysiakini*, April 17, 2020. https://www.malaysiakini.com/news/521057.

Fa Abdul. 2020. "Makcik Kiah must be very disappointed." *Malaysiakini*, August 12, 2020. https://www.malaysiakini.com/columns/538366.

Faisal Asyraf. 2021. "Wrong to fine one-year old child for not wearing mask, chides minister." *Malaysiakini*, February 25, 2021. https://www.malaysiakini.com/news/564369.

Ibrahim Ali. 2020. "SURAT | Buat SOP biarlah masuk akal [Make an SOP that makes sense]." *Malaysiakini*, November 25, 2020. https://www.malaysiakini.com/letters/552515.

Lee, Annabelle, and Mohd Hariz. 2020. "Dazed and confused: Covid-19 positive patients wait at home in limbo", December 30, 2020. https://www.malaysiakini.com/news/557037.

Lee Boon Chye. 2020. "MP speaks | Face mask policy must be clear, without ambiguities." *Malaysiakini*, August 6, 2020. https://www.malaysiakini.com/news/537573.

Low, Choon Chyuan. 2021. "MCO conundrum. 'He kept begging to move in. What were we to do?'" *Malaysiakini*, February 3, 2021. https://www.malaysiakini.com/news/561511.

M Fakrul Halim. 2021. "Physical SPM classes end on Feb 9, Maszlee urges minister to explain why." *Malaysiakini*, February 7, 2021. https://www.malaysiakini.com/news/562014.

Malaysiakini. 2020a. " 'Confusing instructions' – Amanah Youth asks what PM and ministers doing." March 18, 2020. https://www.malaysiakini.com/news/515233.

Malaysiakini. 2020b. "Anwar urges gov't to provide complete info to lessen panic." March 18, 2020. https://www.malaysiakini.com/news/515216.

Malaysiakini. 2020c. "Yoursay: PM, we may have lost Covid-19 battle even before it started." March 20, 2020. https://www.malaysiakini.com/news/515618.

Malaysiakini. 2020d. "Only head of family allowed out for daily essentials, says senior minister." March 21, 2020. https://www.malaysiakini.com/news/515875.

Malaysiakini. 2020e. "Freight forwarders cry foul over contradictory instructions." 22March 2020. https://www.malaysiakini.com/news/516304.

Malaysiakini. 2020f. "Groups say gov't's fake news awareness alert 'unclear, confusing." April 11, 2020. https://www.malaysiakini.com/news/520068.

Malaysiakini. 2020g. "Putrajaya freezes MM2H applications, leaving agents confused." July 2, 2020. https://www.malaysiakini.com/news/532682.

Malaysiakini. 2020h. "Confused? Here's where and when to wear face masks." August 5, 2020. https://www.malaysiakini.com/news/537407.

Malaysiakini. 2020i. "DAP MPs criticise Putrajaya for confusion over work-from-home SOPs." October 22, 2020. https://www.malaysiakini.com/news/547563.

Malaysiakini. 2020j. "Ismail Sabri chuckles over confusion on 'work from home' SOPs." October 21, 2020. https://www.malaysiakini.com/news/547521.

Malaysiakini. 2020k. "Ismail sidesteps Yeoh's criticism, says people need to know actions taken." October 22, 2020. https://www.malaysiakini.com/letters/547656.

Malaysiakini. 2020l. "Families not allowed to circumvent 'two per household' rule in multiple vehicles." November 10, 2020. https://www.malaysiakini.com/news/550319.

Malaysiakini. 2020m. "Confusion over CMCO rules and other news you may have missed." November 11, 2020. https://www.malaysiakini.com/news/550368.

Malaysiakini. 2021g. "Viral video of crammed MAEPS quarantine centre misleading – Nadma." January 9, 2021. https://www.malaysiakini.com/news/558284.

Malaysiakini. 2021h. "MCO 2.0 – what you can and can't do this time." January 13, 2021. https://www.malaysiakini.com/news/558704.

Malaysiakini. 2021i. "New MCO 2.0 rules: a guide to what's changed", January 30, 2021. https://www.malaysiakini.com/news/560983.

Malaysiakini. 2021j. "MMA blasts blame game over Covid-19 cases, wants apology." January 31, 2021. https://www.malaysiakini.com/news/561106.

Malaysiakini. 2021k. "MP: Instil greater awareness, not stiffer penalties to deal with Covid-19." February 1, 2021. https://www.malaysiakini.com/news/561270.

Malaysiakini. 2021l. "Confused and upset, politicians want new SOP for Chinese New Year." February 5, 2021. https://www.malaysiakini.com/news/561767.

Malaysiakini. 2021m. "Unity Ministry seeks review of SOP of Chinese New Year SOP celebrations." February 5, 2021. https://www.malaysiakini.com/news/561827.

Malaysiakini. 2021n. "Hua Zong denies taking part in talks with govt on CNY ruling." February 5, 2021. https://www.malaysiakini.com/news/561867.

Malaysiakini. 2021o. "Upcoming SPM exams need clear SOP early – educator." February 6, 2021. https://www.www.malaysiakini.com/news/561989.

Malaysiakini. 2021p. "Top cop concedes that enforcers find MCO SOPs confusing." February 8, 2021. https://www.malaysiakini.com/news/562045.

Malaysiakini. 2021q. "Daim: PN fails to instil confidence with confusing policies." February 15, 2021. https://www.malaysiakini.com/news/562971.

Malaysiakini. 2021r. "SOP violation: Minister says cops to decide, no need for DAP's judgment." February 16, 2021. https://www.malaysiakini.com/news/563153.

Malaysiakini. 2021s. "Interdistrict travel fine: Minister explains confusion." February 23, 2021. https://www.malaysiakini.com/news/564062.

Malaysiakini. 2021t. "MCO: Stiffer penalties and warrantless arrests under emergency rules." February 28, 2021. https://www.malaysiakini.com/news/564394.

Malaysiakini. 2021u. "RM10k fine fiasco." March 15, 2021. https://www.malaysiakini.com/newsletter/566586.

Malaysiakini. 2021v. "SURAT | Covid-19: Usah terhantuk baru tengadah [LETTER | Covid 19: Look up before getting hit]." January 2, 2021. https://www.malaysiakini.com/letters/557337.

Mohammad Firdaus Low Abdullah. 2020. "LETTER | Tackling the fake news pandemic." May 15, 2020. https://www.malaysiakini.com/letters/525769.

Oh, Steve. 2021. "Emergency puts democracy into an induced coma," *Malaysiakini*, January 29, 2021. https://www.malaysiakini.com/columns/560854.

Raj, JS. 2020. "LETTER | Political ping pong amidst a pandemic." *Malaysiakini*, October 18, 2020. https://www.malaysiakini.com/letters/547004.

Ramieza Wahid. 2020. "Confusion leads Klang residents to police station for travel permission." *Malaysiakini*, October 8, 2020. https://www.malaysiakini.com/news/545806.

Ramieza Wahid. 2021a. "Ex-patient: Social stigma more painful than Covid-19." *Malaysiakini*, January 6, 2021. https://www.malaysiakini.com/news/557795.

Ramieza Wahid. 2021b. "Standardise MCO SOPs for all festivals, says Terengganu PKR chief." Malaysiakini, February 6, 2021. https://www.malaysiakini.com/news/561974.

Reuters/Malaysiakini. 2020. "Explainer: How does AstraZeneca's vaccine compare with Pfizer-BioNTech?" December 31, 2020. https://www.malaysiakini.com/news/557094.

Surin, Jacqueline Ann. 2020. "Surviving the MCO and beyond." *Malaysiakini*, April 28, 2020. https://www.malaysiakini.com/columns/522872.

Tan, KK, and Anshar Azmi. 2021. "COMMENT | Snap general election not needed to change govt." *Malaysiakini*, January 7, 2021. https://www.malaysiakini.com/columns/557976.

Tan, Nathaniel. 2020. "COMMENT | We need clarity, not confusion and red tape." *Malaysiakini*, November 14, 2020. https://www.malaysiakini.com/columns/550879.

Tong, Geraldine. 2020. "Is MCO necessary? Other countries didn't resort to lockdown, says Jomo." *Malaysiakini*, November 15, 2020. https://www.malaysiakini.com/news/550967.

Welsh, Bridget. 2020. "COMMENT | The unsung role of state gov'ts in battling Covid." *Malaysiakini*, July 3, 2020. https://www.malaysiakini.com/columns/532836.

Yi Rong Hoo, Billy. 2020. "Detention centres poised to form coronavirus clusters." *Malaysiakini*, April 23, 2020. https://www.malaysiakini.com/news/522111.

CHAPTER 9

Taiwan Inside and Out:
Redefining the Self during the Pandemic

Craig A Smith & Dayton Lekner

Abstract

This chapter examines how one of the key binaries of Chinese thought—that of *nei–wai* (internal–external)—has evolved during the COVID-19 pandemic in Taiwan and is reflected in its discourses on its neighbours. The authors argue that the pandemic has served as a meta-catalyst in which material and discursive conditions continue to transform the way that Taiwanese construct and understand their identity and their world.

Keywords: Taiwan, migrant workers, New Southbound Policy, *nei-wai*

The pandemic which began in 2020 set in motion a series of disruptions, or departures from the norm, rendering exceptional aspects of lives which were previously quotidian, and rendering mundane those which were previously novel. To cross a border became a distant memory, while to work from home shifted from novelty to necessity, and then monotony. More crucially, to hear of illness or even death in a neighbouring area or country became not a reason to mourn but a metric by which progress or its lack was marked.

Taiwan itself is a state of exceptions. Although a self-governed and democratic island of 23 million, it is excepted from the contemporary global community which takes the nation-state as a basic unit and building block. Governed by the Japanese from 1895 to 1945, Taiwan was then transferred to the Republic of China (ROC) after World War II. The ROC, a state centred around the person of Chiang Kai-shek, then retreated to its newly acquired island in 1949 after defeat in a civil war with Communist forces. Chiang and his own forces established a China under martial law, an alternative to Mao Zedong's PRC. This repressive state evolved, through much internal struggle and external pressure, into a fledging, and soon fully formed and highly transparent democracy. However, despite its comparatively liberal political situation, Taiwan remains unrecognised as a sovereign state by all but a handful of nations.

This journey has left the Taiwanese people with some exceptions of their own. The threat of invasion by the People's Republic of China has created a cognitive dissonance for the citizenry. Taiwan is at once an heir of traditional Chinese culture and a society in need of protection from the contemporary Chinese state. This has led to a continuous—and continuously self-censored—rearticulation of Taiwan's ontology, a redefining of itself and other, or its internal and external.

The relationship between those considered internal and those considered external is central to any community, but it has a particular heritage in the Chinese language. 内–外[*Nei–wai*] (internal–external) is one of the key dyads in Chinese thought and a popular binary through which some of China's most distinguished scholars of intellectual history have understood historical change. In his magnum opus *The Rise of Modern Chinese Thought*, Wang Hui (2014) explains that the eighteenth and nineteenth centuries saw a transition from views of the world as all encompassed by 天下 [*Tianxia*] (all under heaven), to which there was no external 天下無外 [*tianxia wu wai*], to one in which China became one amongst other states and entered into the Westphalian system and an episteme founded on foreign affairs, a reification of the very idea of externality. *Tianxia*, in which all is internal, had met the edges of a system of states which made externality a key to apprehending the world. More recently, Ge Zhaoguang has argued that changing attitudes to the *nei* and *wai* of China have defined self–other binaries throughout China's history and should therefore play an important role in any definition of China (Ge, 2017). These scholars have encouraged consideration of China's past and present relationships with Korea, Japan, and other countries. But Taiwan's self–other binary remains a more complicated problem for such studies.

Despite Taiwan's political ostracisation, its growing economic might has led to the complicated position of a sub-empire. Chen Kuan-hsing has criticised Taiwan's 南向政策 [*nanxiang zhengce*] (Southern Policy), an economic plan which saw factories built in other Asian countries beginning in the 1990s, as an example of the colonised's adoption of the coloniser's historical perspective, as Taiwan's state and society have often identified with Japanese and Western imperialists (Chen, 2010). Long a victim of both Western and Eastern empires, Taiwan plays a sub-imperialist role in Asia today, although this role is quite different from those played by middle power countries such as Canada and Australia. Pride in the exportation of capital to Southeast Asia has helped to enforce attitudes of superiority, which were only further enforced in 2020 with intense pride over Taiwan's early handling of the pandemic. Although the 新南向政策 [*xin nanxiang zhengce*] (New Southbound Policy) under Tsai Ing-wen has proposed a more cooperative alternative to early expansionist visions, these sentiments are deeply ingrained and colour Taiwanese understandings of neighbouring countries, particularly during the pandemic.

This chapter examines Taiwan's shifting views of the internal and external by considering Taiwanese discourse on its neighbours during the pandemic. We argue that the pandemic served as a sort of meta-catalyst, by which both material and discursive conditions were at once brought to light and altered, transforming the way Taiwanese understand their nation and their world. We conclude that while the ever-important Taiwan–China relations continue to shape the construction of Taiwanese identity, the discourse in traditional and social media during the pandemic exposed a dynamic constellation of points by which Taiwan's people triangulate their place in the world and thus their own identity. As Taiwanese pride leads to a reappraisal of those within and without the country's borders, Taiwan's place in Asia, as well as the composition of its internal and its external, are being redefined.

1. Taiwan's Response to the Pandemic

The internal–external dyad shaped the first year of the pandemic from the outset with the presidential election held on January 11, 2020. Despite ongoing domestic concerns regarding labour rights, housing affordability, and environmental protection, the campaign was largely fought and won on the issue of Taiwan's relationship with the PRC, with incumbent Tsai Ing-wen representing distance from the neighbouring world power. Prior to election day, that relationship came into even sharper relief when, from December 31, 2019, reports of atypical pneumonia in Wuhan reached the Taiwan Centres for Disease Control (CDC) (Su and Han, 2020). The CDC, in conjunction with the Central Epidemic Command Centre (CECC), then led a response, initiating immediate screening of all passengers arriving from Wuhan weeks ahead of most of the world. Screening was then expanded to all from "high-risk" areas from late January, and then to all crossing the border in early February. By mid-March, entry was restricted for all except Taiwanese citizens, residents, and certain visa-holders (Summers et al., 2020). This external and geographical perimeter was then bolstered with an internal and temporal equivalent. Legislation established in the wake of the 2003 SARS outbreak enabled the linking of individuals' travel history with their National Health Insurance (NHI) card, alerting medical workers to potential cases. Additionally, returnees were required to quarantine at home for fourteen days, during which they would be monitored via a combination of SMS messages, calls, and a smart-phone app (Summers et al., 2020).

As would occur globally over the following months, these measures largely isolated Taiwan, creating a 本土防綫 [bentu fangxian] (native perimeter). In Taiwan's case, despite its proximity to the centre of the outbreak and extensive familial, touristic, and economic links with the mainland, the perimeter was so successful that it created a space within, in which cases were falling rapidly to zero, and a world without, in which they were rising exponentially. It was no surprise, therefore, that print, digital, and social media discussion focused on what led to the outbreak and to failures in its containment. At first, such discussion shared with the presidential campaign both the fear and othering of the Chinese people and their government. While many scholars have rightly been critical of Western "Sinophobic" readings of the outbreak (Roche, 2020; Smith, 2020), similar stereotyping discourse continues to be widespread in Taiwan. Television news initially ran stories about bat-eating locals in Wuhan, and print and digital media repeated what had begun as Shanghai- and Beijing-based stereotyping of Wuhanese as reflecting the cultural practices of all mainland Chinese (*Apple Daily*, January 23, 2020). As Liu Shao-hua has pointed out, even the naming of the virus in Taiwan exhibited an othering of the mainland (Liu, 2020). As an explanation for global and racialised or culturally essentialising discourse, "Sinophobia" fails to explain this "othering" *within* the Sinosphere. Rather, the internal–external division acts as a more foundational epistemic practice which can be applied both within and without the vastly complex and variegated world of Chinese culture and language, and operates simultaneously at levels of race, culture, nation, and locality.

Simultaneous to this cultural othering of those at the centre of the outbreak was a political othering of their state. The spectre of CPC authoritarianism, omnipresent in Taiwan but highlighted during the election campaign, provided another clear point of reference outside the Taiwanese national identity. Lockdowns, media blackouts, and a lack of transparency within Wuhan and across the mainland were all covered heavily in Taiwanese media. These have been dominant also in English language media and thus will not be rehashed here. We simply note that, in its opening stages, the pandemic acted to intensify predominant and polar views of Taiwan–China relations along the *nei–wai* axis.

2. Rethinking Taiwan's External

The pandemic augmented this cross-strait Janus construction of the internal and external, complicating the notion of what it meant to be or not be Taiwanese. From March, a growing list of nations and cultures proved permeable to the virus, each in turn prompting discussion within Taiwan about the reasons for their failures. The rapidly shifting focus of fear of the external, and its epistemic partner, chauvinism, even in real-time required daily reading to keep up with, and in relaying it here we approach the infamous Lenny Bruce stand-up routine in which all present are treated to a personalised racist epithet. The Japanese were devoted to work (敬業的精神 [*jingye de jingshen*]) and lacked 敵意 [*diyi*] (hostility) towards China (*Liberty Times*, February 16, 2020). Iran was dominated by a fanatical clergy, folk beliefs

(*Mirror Media*, May 12, 2020), and folk habits (*Liberty Times*, March 17, 2020), and led by an Ayatollah duped by PRC propaganda (*Mirror Media*, May 17, 2020). Italians, by March the worst affected nation in Europe, were a 樂天民族 [*letian minzu*] (carefree people) consumed by an interest in spaghetti (Jiang, 2020), and weakened against the virus by a culturally embedded 小聰明 [*xiao congming*] (craftiness), through which they found ways to shirk restrictions (*Central News Agency*, March 9, 2020).

These roving and casual caricatures unearthed the sort of cultural stereotyping which occurred globally and were brought into relief by the pandemic as media organisations and individuals struggled to understand the spread of the virus. In this, Taiwan was far from unique. However, Taiwan's status as quasi-nation-state adds an exceptional element to this phenomenon and process. In the years leading into the pandemic, Taiwan had been seeking representation as either member state or even observer at the World Health Organization (WHO). In the opening months of 2020, Taiwan made numerous attempts to informally participate in the WHO response to the pandemic. The WHO however, under the leadership of Tedros Adhanom Ghebreyesus, and requiring the cooperation of the PRC—which steadfastly refused to admit Taiwan in any capacity—continued to exclude Taiwan from global discussion on the pandemic (Yin, 2021). This situation came to a head in April 2020, when Tedros accused Taiwan of racist attacks against his person, triggering a terse response from the Taiwanese foreign ministry, and anger in online bulletin boards and on YouTube (Lin, 2020). The overall effect, however, beyond these explanations which perhaps raised more questions than they answered, was a near ubiquitous disillusionment with the international body, into which Taiwan had so desperately sought entrée. Thus, when American president Donald Trump ramped up his own attacks on the WHO and signalled his own intention to remove the U.S. from the body, many in Taiwan read the move as Taiwan and the United States standing united against a corrupt global system dominated by the PRC (*Commonwealth Magazine*, April 9, 2020).

Again, the internal–external dyad helps us think through these ruptures and sutures. We can see the Westphalian system of states as a successor to China's *tianxia* model, as now all recognised states are internal to the global body. Taiwan's forced externality to this community resulted in an increasing sense of being isolated and silenced in a year in which states were both increasingly balkanised through border closures, and increasingly reliant on shared information in their fight against COVID-19. That Tedros counterattacked demands for Taiwan's inclusion by presenting the Taiwanese as racist, resulted, perhaps foreseeably, in genuine anger in Taiwanese media and online discussion. When Trump acted to limit U.S. engagement with the WHO, Taiwanese people felt a degree of relief, bolstering support for the maverick American president. Trump's actions and rhetoric thus acknowledged and drew attention to a position outside the global internal—explicating a space in which Taiwan had long existed and rendering it not only real, but globally recognised. This then fed back into a domestic discourse which was ever more aware of Taiwan's success in controlling COVID-19, a success which was not only achieved while external to the global community, but which was to a degree founded on that externality. This created not only an acceptance of Taiwan's externality to a global other, but a conscious explication and even celebration of that externality. In 2020, for the first time in recent history, the Taiwanese found a path to nationalism not in spite of, but based upon, their own exceptional situation. However, this is only half the story, as while Taiwanese identity vis-à-vis the external global was being redrawn, so was its internal counterpart.

3. Rethinking Taiwan's Internal

In 2020, the first year of the pandemic, illegal migrant workers tested positive for COVID-19, highlighting their precarious position in Taiwan's society and presenting an opportunity for further consideration of the *nei–wai* binary and changing understandings of Taiwan's internal and external (Ho, 2020). In the Chinese language, 外勞 [*wai-lao*] or "foreign labourer" has long been used to indicate the many workers coming from Southeast Asia and other areas. However, in recent years, although the term *wai-lao* has remained common in other Sinophone communities, Taiwan has increasingly turned to the word 移工 [*yi-gong*] (migrant worker). Much like the term 老外 [*lao-wai*] (foreigner or westerner) in different contexts, *wai-lao* is now often seen as discriminatory language.

The crisis of the pandemic concentrated focus upon the plight of migrant workers in different ways. In 2020, establishing exactly who should be regarded as internal became an important matter for state and society, as the marginalised became further marginalised. States hurried to provide support to citizens and workers, while in many countries foreigners and those in the gig economy or working illegally found themselves unable to access support packages. This was certainly true in Taiwan, where massive networks of foreign labourers and caregivers are employed, often for extended periods but with limited labour rights.

Migrant workers play crucial roles in Taiwan labour, with most from Southeast Asian nations, including Indonesia, Thailand, and the Philippines. In 1992, Taiwan's government introduced the Employment Services Act, allowing the employ of migrant workers to stop the outflow of capital to Southeast Asia (Hoang, 2017). At the same time, under the Kuomintang president Lee Teng-hui, the government had been actively pursuing the exportation of financial capital to Southeast Asian countries through the Southern Policy, a collection of 1990s institutions aimed at economic expansion along a discursive and political trajectory which mirrored

Japanese efforts from one hundred years earlier. The acceleration of the reform and opening up of China redirected financial capital to the PRC in the decades following Lee's rule, but the Tsai government returned to these ideas with the New Southbound Policy as part of her 2016 campaign promise to lessen economic dependence on China. Once again, Southeast Asian countries are the focus of Taiwan's policies, but the social conditions of Taiwan in the pandemic are markedly different from Taiwan in the 1990s.

The number of migrants has steadily increased over the past three decades and approximately 700,000 were living in Taiwan in 2021. Although this number pales in comparison with Japan's, which is more than twice that, Taiwan's population remains under 24 million, indicating that documented migrant workers now total approximately three per cent of the population, slightly larger than the number of officially recognised indigenous people (Republic of China National Statistics, 2021). However, beginning in early 2020, restrictions limited the number of labourers coming from these countries and created difficulties for many wanting to return. In December, migrant workers from Indonesia were no longer allowed entry after hundreds tested positive for COVID-19 on arrival.

The Ministry of Labor releases an annual report on migrant workers every January. The "Statistical Results from the 2020 Investigation into the Management and Utilization of Migrant Workers" was released in January 2021. According to the report, the average monthly salary for legal migrant workers in June 2020 was NT$28,583 (US$1,000), while the average salary for migrant care workers in June was only 19,918, including 2,075 from overtime hours and based on an average workday of 10.1 to 10.5 hours. While the wages earned from overtime have increased, the caretakers' total salary reflects a slight decrease from the previous two years (Ministry of Labor, 2021). In January 2021, Taiwan's minimum salary for full-time workers was raised from 23,100 to 23,800, but migrant workers do not qualify for most of the protections offered by the Ministry of Labor.

Even before the pandemic, these workers were marginalised, with frequent reports of abuse and even strict controls over women's fertility, prompting many to escape from their employers and find other means of making a living (Cheng, 2020). Of the already-marginalised migrant workers in Taiwan, thousands disappear every year. Lan Anh Hoang has pointed out that this trend for Vietnamese workers, who are the worst violators of visa regulations, was 8.66% at the end of 2012 (Hoang, 2017). In November 2016, the National Immigration Agency estimated that 53,801 migrant workers were missing (Han, 2017). By the end of 2020, despite fewer migrant workers residing in Taiwan during the pandemic, this number was not very different at 52,000 (Xiao, 2020).

As it became all but impossible to repatriate foreign workers during the pandemic, detention centres were overflowing in 2020 and 2021. Many migrants were unable to afford air tickets, which in 2020 became up to four times as expensive as they once were. These migrants simply turned themselves over to government detention centres at the end of their contract. With nowhere for these illegal migrants to be housed, most were immediately released, and the government was soon no longer willing to expend resources tracking down and arresting them. However, illegal migrants released into society were still unable to legally enter employment. The authorities were well aware that the migrants had no choice but to enter illegal labour markets (Xiao, 2020).

This resulted in an increased subalternisation of illegal migrant workers. They proceeded from an already precarious position in which they had reduced access to government support to one in which they had no legal recourse at all. At the same time, from the government's perspective, this presented a gap in the nation's defence against the pandemic. Undocumented migrants remained outside of information networks. They had no access to health networks and testing. And their poverty often reduced their willingness to purchase masks or other preventative products, such as hand sanitiser, which became ubiquitous in the rest of society (Chen, 2020).

Once Taiwan's "native perimeter" first collapsed in 2021 and the virus raced across urban areas, marginalised people were targeted. Although sex workers and their clients were initially blamed in news reports on rising cases in a popular red-light district, migrant workers were also forced into the spotlight again. After outbreaks at technology factories, in which the majority of infected workers were migrant workers living in dormitories, the Miaoli County government prohibited all migrant workers from leaving their residences. The responsibility for enforcing this law often fell to employers, who were subject to heavy fines of NT$60,000 to 300,000 In turn, some employers were reported to have illegally forced migrants to sign forms indicating they would bear the full medical costs of any COVID-19 infection (Everington, 2021).

The contradiction of these migrants living In Taiwan while remaining external to Taiwan's support networks was exacerbated and illuminated during the pandemic, but there were positive responses. NGOs, such as the Taiwan International Workers' Association (TIWA tiwa.org.tw) have long played a role in organising workers and have continued to fight for human rights throughout the pandemic. Near the end of 2020, TIWA issued three demands for the rights of migrant workers:

1. The government must bear the costs of quarantine and must promise to improve the conditions of the dormitories used for migrants during their quarantine and while they are working.

2. The government must face up to the demands of Taiwan's long-term carers and ensure that migrant domestic workers are seen as part of the long-term-carer workforce and are covered by guaranteed working conditions.

3. The government must bear the responsibility of recruitment and placement through government-to-government links, and it must bring an end to private recruitment agencies (Xie, 2020).

The TIWA has performed a leading role in representing migrant workers and opposing restrictions, including the fight against the Miaoli crackdowns (Wu, 2021). The organisation opposes all labour hierarchies, arguing that all those working in Taiwan should be treated equally, even to the extent that migrant workers should have the right to vote on any policies which will affect them (Taiwan International Workers' Association, 2021).

Although similar issues with migrant workers have troubled Taiwan for decades, as with the ongoing issue of Taiwan's relationship with China, these issues were brought to the forefront during the pandemic, and we witnessed an acceleration of identity formation as material and discursive changes forced a reconceptualisation of Taiwan inside and out.

4. Conclusion: "Taiwan Helps Asia, and Asia Helps Taiwan"

The pandemic dramatically changed the self-image of Taiwanese and further cemented a Taiwanese identity independent of China and increasingly independent of the global system of states. This change was a disruption to long-running hesitation and ambiguity towards Taiwan's identity formation. It accelerated the process and further united the population through the othering of Taiwan's external. With the onset of the pandemic in early 2020, critics of China jumped at the opportunity to depict the country as unclean and barbaric, defining Taiwan through contradistinction. This self-definition was reinforced throughout 2020, as Western countries in particular bungled responses to the pandemic and an unprecedented expression of *Taiwanness* was formulated after the first year of the pandemic. This was an expression which was fuelled by an increasing awareness, and even celebration, of Taiwan's externality to a global community. In January 2021, taking advantage of the tremendous pride in Taiwan related to the pandemic response, the government announced a new passport which removed the English title "Republic of China," the official name of the country, from the cover. This was a strong statement to the external world, demanding discursive inclusion in the world community as Taiwan. Chinese characters on the cover continued to use the name Republic of China, but this mixed messaging was a clear representation of rising Taiwanese nationalism, and of the plural and interlocking edges of the internal–external borders which Taiwan must manage to express this nationalism.

Within this exceptional nationalism, an equal complexity of margins and marginalised prevails, as migrant workers with limited formal rights struggle for representation in the national community. The continued marginalisation of migrant workers as external ensures Taiwanese superiority through this neoliberal system of governance, but such an internal hierarchy is in stark contradiction with the promotion of Taiwan's foreign policy. Taiwan must walk a careful line to ensure that the New Southbound Policy does not engage in a re-establishment of traditional colonial hierarchies as the country strives to leave China and join the nations of Asia. The policy is promoted through the slogan of "Taiwan Helps Asia, and Asia Helps Taiwan," an exclamation of a 人為核心 [*ren wei hexin*] (people-centred) movement, but the disconnect between discourse and practice has become evident as Southeast Asian migrant workers are consistently identified as outsiders during the pandemic (Ministry of Trade, 2021).

Thus, Taiwan within and without represents a multi-layered struggle for recognition, and a jostle between the internal and external as nationalism is recalibrated and reassessed. Intense feelings of pride distinguished the Taiwanese pandemic experience from the rest of the world's, and these feelings continue to influence Taiwan's defining of its internal and external. Taiwan's particular history and place in contemporary geopolitics make unique its experience of the pandemic which began in 2020. But these characteristics also render more vivid aspects of experience shared by nations and peoples globally. The pandemic has catalysed both waves of xenophobia and a redrawing and enhancing of *nei–wei* divisions. It has also forced both state and individual re-evaluation of the domestic, foreign, and border policies which define each country's *nei–wai* relations and, with these, what it means to be a member of that modern entity, the national imagined community. As with other periods of disruption (most obviously found in wartime), the augmented sense of a divide between the internal and external is accompanied, somewhat paradoxically, by a narrowing of differences as each nation deals, in increased isolation, with a shared threat. We suggest here that the *nei–wai* dyad is important for its ability to call attention to our increased isolation and the need to overcome it.

Craig A. Smith is Senior Lecturer of Translation Studies at the University of Melbourne's Asia Institute. He is a historian of modern China and an avid translator. His publications include *Chinese Asianism* (Harvard University Asia Center, 2021) and the co-edited *Translating the Occupation: The Japanese Invasion of China* (UBC, 2021).

Dayton Lekner writes and translates histories of 20th century China. His work has appeared in *Modern China, Twentieth Century China, The Journal of Asian Studies*, and *Contemporary Chinese Thought*. He holds a PhD from the University of Melbourne (2019) and an MA from National Taiwan University (2015).

References

Apple Daily. 2020. "E! Zhongguoren chi bianfu yingpian baoguang." [Ew! Video of Chinese people eating bats exposed]. January 23, 2020. https://tw.appledaily.com/international/20200123/WAT7R-JS3ZOUCSWPGM3GCAUZS5I/.

Central News Agency. 2020. "Yidali beibu da fengcheng dan fangyi nan leguan: 'Women chengle xin Wuhan.'" [Northern Italy is locked down but no room for optimism in epidemic prevention 'we are the new Wuhan']. March 9, 2020. https://www.cna.com.tw/news/firstnews/202003090170.aspx.

Chen, Hantang. 2020. "Feiyan kunjingxia de yigong jiaolv." [Migrant worker anxiety under pandemic dilemma]. *Duli Pinglun.* March 14, 2020. https://opinion.cw.com.tw/blog/profile/52/article/9182

Chen, Kuan-hsing. 2010. *Asia as Method: Toward Deimperialization.* Durham and London: Duke University Press.

Cheng, Isabelle. 2020. "We want productive workers, not fertile women." *Asia Pacific Viewpoint* 61, no. 3: 453–465.

Commonwealth Magazine. 2020. "Yu Tan Desai zuodui 'Meilianshe:' Meiguo liyong yiqing tisheng Taiwan guoji diwei." [The Associated Press stands against Tedros: United States uses the pandemic to enhance Taiwan's international status]. April 9, 2020. https://www.cw.com.tw/article/5099792.

Everington, Keoni. 2021. "21 migrant workers in Miaoli questioned by police for venturing out." *Taiwan News.* June 9, 2021. https://www.taiwannews.com.tw/en/news/4219019?fbclid=IwAR1J9xlZo-hgp3Et-vC5yyWi-rbI26hfK33fQSh9zSioqwJMTRWw6QtBZAQU.

Ge, Zhaoguang. 2017. *Lishi Zhongguo de nei yu wai* [Nei and Wai in Historical China]. Hong Kong: Chinese University of Hong Kong Press.

Han, Peijie. 2017. "Quxiao yigong sannian xu chujing yiri yu shilian yigong renshu zhang zhi guan-lianxing." [The connection between cancellation of need for migrant workers to leave the country at least one day in every three years and increase in numbers of missing workers]. *National Immigration Agency.* https://www.immigration.gov.tw/media/5988/%E5%8F%96%E6%B6%88%E7%A7%BB%E5%B7%A5%E4%B8%89%E5%B9%B4%E9%A0%88%E5%87%BA%E5%A2%83%E4%B8%80%E6%97%A5%E8%88%87%E5%A4%B1%E8%81%AF%E7%A7%BB%E5%B7%A5%E4%BA%BA%E6%95%B8%E6%88%90%E9%95%B7%E4%B9%8B%E9%97%9C%E8%81%AF%E6%80%A7.pdf.

Ho, Ming-sho. 2020. "Watchdogs and partners: Taiwan's civil society organizations." *Carnegie Europe.* December 7, 2020. https://carnegieeurope.eu/2020/12/07/watchdogs-and-partners-taiwan-s-civil-so-ciety-organizations-pub-83140?fbclid=IwARomkzQ6HQ7iJCWDaFBjvEqn5NhSF7WfBokfys2lkI5Ul-qlQjz7PlwqtFb4.

Hoang, Lan Anh. 2017. "Governmentality in Asian migration regimes: The case of labour migration from Vietnam to Taiwan." *Population, Space and Place* 23, no. 3: 1–12. https://www.mirrormedia.mg/story/20200512edi023/.

Jiang, Xinghan. 2020. "Yaoyuan youru xinguanbingdu! Yiguo Tairen: Yidali dengyu Wuhan kong yanguoqishi." [Rumours spread like the virus! Taiwanese in Italy: To say Italy is like Wuhan is an exaggeration]. *Global News Monthly.* March 13, 2020. https://www.gvm.com.tw/article/71574.

Liberty Times. 2020. "Dai kouzhao wufa xihu! Yilangren jie dangdi yiqing baofa guanjian yuanyin." [Can't breath with a mask on! Iranians reveal root of local outbreak]. March 17, 2020. https://ent.ltn.com.tw/news/breakingnews/3103147.

Liberty Times. 2020. "Wuhan feiyan: Taiwan fangyi weihe lingxian Riben? Xiangmin 8dian fenxi bei tuibao." [Wuhan Pneumonia – Why is Taiwan's epidemic prevention ahead of Japan's? Netizens' 8-point analysis tweeted widely]. February 16, 2020. https://news.ltn.com.tw/news/politics/break-ingnews/3069564.

Lin, Vivi. 2020. "An Open Letter to Dr. Tedros." YouTube video. Accessed March 25, 2021. https://youtu.be/EKh6qiAGDfA.

Liu, Shao-hua. 2020. "Feiyan yiqingxia tan jibing de mingming yu wuming." [On names and stigma in the pandemic]. *Duli Pinglun*. March 4, 2020. https://opinion.cw.com.tw/blog/profile/406/article/9150. For English translation, see https://www.readingthechinadream.com/liu-shao-hua-disease-names-and-stigma.html.

Ministry of Labor. 2021. *109nian yigong guanli ji yunyong diaocha tongji jieguo 109* [Statistical Results of 2020 migrant worker management and utilization survey]. https://www.mol.gov.tw/media/90 36589/109%E5%B9%B4%E7%A7%BB%E5%B7%A5%E7%AE%A1%E7%90%86%E5%8F%8A%E9% 81%8B%E7%94%A8%E8%AA%BF%E6%9F%A5%E7%B5%B1%E8%A8%88%E7%B5%90%E6%9E %9C-%E5%90%AB%E5%9C%96%E8%A1%A8.pdf.

Ministry of Trade. 2021. *New Southbound Policy Implementation Plans*. https://newsouthboundpolicy.trade.gov.tw/English/PageDetail?pageID=49&nodeID=94.

Mirror Media. 2020. "Jingyou tu gangmeng: Zhi Wuhan feiyan? Yilangren tingxin pianfang yiqing jiaju." [Essential oils on the anus to treat Wuhan flu? Epidemic intensifies as Iranians follow folk remedies]. May 12, 2020. https://www.mirrormedia.mg/story/20200512edi023/.

Republic of China National Statistics. 2021. Accessed March 25, 2021. http://statdb.dgbas.gov.tw/.

Roche, Gerald. 2020. "The epidemiology of sinophobia." *Made in China Journal*, January–April, 2020. https://madeinchinajournal.com/2020/02/17/the-epidemiology-of-sinophobia/.

Smith, Aminda. 2020. "Of martyrs and maladies: Some thoughts on the coronavirus." *Positions Politics*, February 13, 2020. https://positionspolitics.org/aminda-smith-of-martyrs-and-maladies-some-thoughts-on-the-coronavirus/.

Su, Sheng-Fang, and Yueh-Ying Han. 2020. "How Taiwan, a non-WHO member, takes actions in response to COVID-19." *Journal of Global Health* 10, no. 1: 1–5.

Summers, Jennifer, Hao-Yuan Cheng, Hsien-Ho Lin, Lucy Telfar Barnard, Amanda Kvalsvig, Nick Wilson, and Michael G. Baker. 2020. "Potential lessons from the Taiwan and New Zealand health responses to the COVID-19 pandemic." *The Lancet Regional Health-Western Pacific* 2020: 100044.

Taiwan International Workers Association. 2021. Accessed March 25, 2021. https://www.tiwa.org.tw/%e7%b5%84%e7%b9%94%e4%bb%8b%e7%b4%b9/tiwa%e7%b0%a1%e4%bb%8b/.

Wang, Hui. 2014. *Xiandai Zhongguo sixiang de xingqi* [The Rise of Modern Chinese Thought]. Beijing: Sanlian shudian.

Wu, Jingru. 2021. "Fandui Miaolixian zhengfu xianzhi yigong waichu." [Oppose the Miaoli County Government Prohibiting Migrant Workers from Going out] *Taiwan International Workers' Association*. June 10, 2021. https://www.tiwa.org.tw/%E3%80%90%E6%96%B0% E8%81%9E%E7%A8%BF%E3%80%91%E5%8F%8D%E5%B0%8D%E8%8B%97%E6%A0%97 %E7%B8%A3%E6%94%BF%E5%BA%9C%E9%99%90%E5%88%B6%E7%A7%BB%E5%B7%- A5%E5%A4%96%E5%87%BA-%E7%B7%9A%E4%B8%8A%E8%A8%98%E8%80%85/.

Xiao, Tingfang. 2020. "Taiwan cheng da heigong tiantang… wufa qiansong huiguo de shilian yigong." [Taiwan now paradise for illegal workers…Why do uncontactable migrant workers who can't be sent home roam the country and even increase their price?] *Taiwan United Daily News*, December 10, 2020. https://udn.com/news/story/6839/5081188.

Xie, Mengying. 2020. "'Guojia conglai mei ba tamen dangren kan!' 108ming yigong quezhen. Mintuan jie zhenzheng 'fangyi pokou." ['The country has never seen them as people!' 108 migrant workers test positive, reveal weak link in epidemic prevention chain]. *Storm Media*, December 10, 2020. https://www.storm.mg/article/3283645?page=3.

Yin, Jason Dean-Chen. 2021. "WHO, COVID-19, and Taiwan as the Ghost Island." *Global Public Health*, February 26, 2021. https://doi.org/10.1080/17441692.2021.1890184.

CHAPTER 10

Linguistic and Cultural Challenges in Chinese Translation of Government COVID-19 Health Information in Australia

Lachlan Thomas-Walters, Suqin Qian & Delia Lin[1]

Abstract

This chapter highlights the complexity of communicating public health information to culturally and linguistically diverse communities. Drawing on translation evaluation reports generated by ninety students of the University of Melbourne's Master of Translation and Interpreting, this chapter surveys and examines the veracity of official health messaging translated and made available to Chinese communities from state and federal government websites during the COVID-19 pandemic. We compare translated written resources on COVID-19 provided by different Australian states and the federal government, focusing on identifying different approaches to and significant linguistic, cultural, and conceptual discrepancies in the Chinese translation. We argue that a coherent and well-informed approach to communication by responsible government bodies through quality translation is essential in times of health emergency.

Keywords: COVID-19 translated resources, culturally and linguistically diverse communities, Chinese translation, government messaging, health communication

1. Introduction

The COVID-19 pandemic has brought with it considerable disruptions and uncertainties, but these have been further exacerbated by linguistic barriers. There has been no shortage of evidence that the novel coronavirus is having a disproportionately high and negative impact on linguistic minority communities around the world. In their statement on the impact of COVID-19 and racial discrimination, the United Nations Committee on the Elimination of Racial Discrimination (CERD) highlights the global evidence that the pandemic continues to disproportionately affect individuals and communities who belong to "national or ethnic, religious and linguistic minorities," concluding that the pandemic has exacerbated social and structural inequalities, discrimination and exclusion (Committee on the

Elimination of Racial Discrimination, 2020). Responses to the virus have varied all over the world, with countries, international organisations, states and local communities enforcing an array of COVID-19 strategies often in conjunction with differing health advice and tailored to the specific circumstances of the region (Amat et al., 2020; Bakir, 2020; Banerjee, 2020; Benítez et al., 2020; Brown, 2020; de Bruijn et al., 2020; Canestrini, 2020; Capano, 2020; Chabibi and Jamallullail, 2020; Chiplunkar and Das, 2021; Christensen and Lægreid, 2020; Civitarese, 2020). The global pandemic has highlighted the importance of recognising linguistic diversity, embracing social inclusion through language, and safeguarding the health and well-being of society by providing accurate and efficient translated health advice.

In Australia, translated resources on COVID-19 are managed by state and federal government departments. In accurately responding to an evolving and ever-changing pandemic and ensuring the maximum safety and well-being of all society, government departments must be decisive and make informed determinations quickly and resolutely. The changing and developing COVID-19 related rules and regulations across state and territory borders have created ongoing confusion and inconsistency for the Australian public (Aldridge, Moon, and Chisholm, 2021; Bamford, 2020).

This chapter surveys and examines the veracity of government translated resources, in particular, official health messaging translated and made available to Chinese communities from state and federal government websites. We compare translated written resources on COVID-19 provided by different Australian states and the federal government, focusing on identifying different approaches to and significant linguistic, cultural, and conceptual discrepancies in the Chinese translations. The purpose of this chapter is not to assess or critique translation quality or list translation errors, but to highlight a lack of multilingual expertise and credibility in the official messaging of urgent health priorities to communities where English is not a first language. To remedy this and minimise misconceptions, we argue that it is important to advance collective and coordinated efforts equipped to navigate cultural and linguistic complexities in producing accurate and high-quality multilingual material and narratives for effective government dissemination during times of public health emergency. More importantly, our research demonstrates the necessity to improve Australia's multilingual capability in general rather than resorting to quick-fix translation services in times of crisis.

2. A Monolingual Conundrum

The successful safeguarding of citizens against COVID-19 transmission requires a united effort amongst the entire population (World Health Organization, 2020). Overcoming the challenges posed by this unprecedented pandemic necessitates widespread community "buy-in" and participation as the decisions of individuals will profoundly damage the safety of the broader society. To ensure people are following government advice and understanding and adhering to all public health information, it is imperative that all members of society, irrespective of their language or cultural background, receive and comprehend accurate and timely information. Piekkari et al. (2021, p. 590) argue that multilingual nations have been relying on a monolingual approach to combatting the virus, noting that "crises also make communication gaps and voids of social meaning painfully visible. COVID-19 is foregrounding the consequences of what it means (not) to have access to knowledge, safety, justice, and voice—and lack of access is often aggravated, if not produced, by language barriers. Exclusion and inequality grow in the shadows of linguistic dominance."

The need for the dissemination of multilingual health advice is notably pressing in Australia where there are over three hundred separately identified languages spoken in homes (Australian Bureau of Statistics, 2017). The Australian federal and state governments must heed the realities of the ethnically diverse jurisdictions and communities which they supposedly represent. For example, the 2016 national census identifies that more than one-fifth (21%) of Australians speak a language other than English at home, and, after English, the next most common languages spoken at home are Mandarin, Arabic, Cantonese, and Vietnamese. The census shows that two-thirds (67%) of the Australian population were born in Australia with nearly half (49%) having either been born overseas or having one or both parents born overseas. Commenting on Australia's linguistic diversity and the challenges of social inclusion, Piller (2014) argues that Australia has long held a "monolingual mindset," where languages are often put into two categories: "English" and "Other." Academics have identified how "the severe limitations of multilingual crisis communication that the COVID-19 crisis has laid bare result from the dominance of English-centric global mass communication, the longstanding devaluation of minoritised languages, and the failure to consider the importance of multilingual repertoires for building trust and resilient communities" (Piller, Zhang, and Li, 2020, p. 503).

Despite Australia having an increasingly multicultural and multilingual population, the laws, rules, and regulations which govern its people remain monolingual and monocultural (Schalley, Guillemin, and Eisenchlas, 2015). The COVID-19 global pandemic serves as a stark reminder of the need for accurate and effective multilingual dissemination of information. The gaps in information to minority and non-English speaking communities have always existed in Australian political and social life (Judicial Commission of New South Wales, 2021). However, within the context of the current pandemic, the need for fast, efficient, and accurate health advice has never before been more pressing and paramount.

3. Research Methods

This chapter first of all draws on translation evaluation reports generated by ninety students of the University of Melbourne's Master of Translation and Interpreting over three semesters, most of whom (approx. 95%) are native speakers of Chinese who have received primary, secondary, or tertiary education in Taiwan or the People's Republic of China, the remaining 5% being native speakers of English fluent in Mandarin Chinese. The reports were submitted as one of their capstone projects in which the students utilised their skills to assess the accuracy and veracity of Chinese translation of COVID-19 health information published on the Victorian (VIC) Government's Coronavirus (COVID-19) and Government of New South Wales (NSW) websites. We use these reports with the students' permission.

The first cohort, consisting of thirty-one students, examined the lockdown information in August 2020, when Melbourne was under Stage 4 restrictions and regional Victoria, Stage 3. Forty-two per cent of the students found the official government translation erroneous, grammatically incoherent, and in general rendering the overall message ineffective. Moreover, six students (19%) with eminently reliable and sophisticated language and translation skills deemed the Victorian Government interpretation to be so incompetent and indifferent to suggest that the translation may have been generated by machine translation software with little or no human input. The remaining 58% of this study's sample found the Government's translation generally acceptable despite obvious, numerous and unacceptable translation mistakes. The second cohort included twenty-eight students, who analysed the vaccine rollout information published on the COVID-19 Victoria website in March 2021. All the students found the Chinese translation acceptable in terms of conveying essential information on vaccine rollout despite failing to take into account the subtle and marked discrepancies in values and concepts. The third cohort, consisting of thirty-two translators-in-training, examined the COVID-19 restrictions extended in NSW published on the NSW Government website on June 26, 2021. All the students believed that the Chinese translation generated by an automated service on the NSW Government website failed to help the government achieve the intended communication purposes during the pandemic due to numerous erroneous translations at semantic, syntactic, and cultural levels.

We treat the students as both translation critics and readers of the Chinese version of the official government information. Their responses provide us with empirical evidence as to how the Chinese communities might respond to the government messaging in Chinese. The students' observations of significant inadequate translation shape the basis for our comparative analysis of Chinese translations on different state and territory government websites. In the following sections we first survey the fast-moving rules and regulations issued in Australia and in particular,

Victoria, to highlight the gap in the volume of information disseminated in English and multiple other languages. We then conduct a textual analysis of key linguistic and cultural discrepancies in the Chinese translations provided by different state and territory governments.

4. COVID-19 and the Fast-Moving Rules and Regulations

The first case of COVID-19 in Australia was recorded on January 25, 2020. Over a month later, the Australian Government published the *Australian Health Sector Emergency Response Plan for Novel Coronavirus (COVID-19)*, outlining the key areas of disease control, including a plan for the communication of consistent, timely, and accurate health advice (Australian Government Department of Health and Aged Care, 2020a). Amongst the recognised challenges facing the successful dissemination of COVID-19 updates were: managing uncertainty, balancing timely information with accuracy, maintaining consistent messaging across states and territories, and creating two-way communication between the government and the public. On March 13, 2020, to better coordinate and streamline Australia's public health response, the government set up a National Cabinet made up of the Prime Minister, state premiers and territory chief ministers (Parliament of Australia, 2020). In its consideration of the need to provide Australia's most vulnerable and at-risk groups with up-to-date health advice, the government wrote: "the need for provision of advice in other languages, at the border, and domestically will also be considered" (Australian Government Department of Health and Aged Care, 2020a, p. 36).

Despite federal support and advice, individual states and territories are responsible for disease prevention, control, and the dissemination of public health advice in their respective jurisdictions (Mclean and Huf, 2020). Under the Australian federal system, state and territory governments are given a broad range of public health and emergency powers to implement public health measures (Nekvapil, Narayan, and Brenker, 2020). The complexity of different control measures across state and territory borders is best reflected in the spate of acts, orders, bills, amendments, rules, regulations, directions, and guidelines enacted to provide the legal basis for the enforcement of extraordinary measures to stop the spread of the virus.

Allman (2020, p. 32) writes how a little over a month after the New South Wales government announced a "State of Emergency," some twenty-four different public orders and legislative amendments were introduced as "freedom of movement disappeared as borders were shut, non-essential travel was banned, and citizens were ordered to stay home other than to carry out limited vital tasks." In Victoria, on March 16, 2020, the government declared a "State of Emergency," giving it the power to "give any other direction that the authorised officer considers is reasonably necessary to protect public health" (Victorian Legislation, 2020). Subsequently, the Victorian Parliament passed the COVID-19 Omnibus (Emergency Measures) Act 2020 (Vic) making numerous amendments to other legislation and creating additional regulatory powers. Utilising the legal frameworks, the Victorian government introduced an armada of Public Directions designed to protect the public and "stop the spread." As of July 2021, the Deputy Chief Health Officer (Communicable Disease) has passed well over two hundred such directions. These significantly changed social freedom and social practice, and imposed heavy fines for non-compliance. Some of the changes included rules and regulations surrounding isolation, workplace safety, travel, stay at home measures, restricting social, religious and community gatherings, aged-care facilities, as well as direct public health measures such as social distancing, the wearing of facial coverings, and testing procedures. The *Restricted Activity Directions*—introduced to control the operation of businesses and limit the spread of COVID-19—underlines the ever-changing and unstable nature of Victorian regulatory measures (see Appendix 1).

As the circumstances surrounding COVID-19 continue to change, it is unsurprising that government directions must quickly adapt. However, the volume of imposed restrictions has caused confusion, uncertainty, and discombobulation, as indiscriminate rules are imposed for certain *"restricted areas," "restricted postcodes," "non-Melbourne," "Metropolitan Melbourne," "Regional Victoria"* residents, as well as targeted responses to certain public housing estates in North Melbourne and Flemington which were put into "hard" lockdown (Victorian Ombudsman, 2020). These extraordinary, undebated, and uncontested measures were so complicated that Melbourne residents living on the same street (yet sharing different postcodes) were subjected to different COVID-19 restrictions (Boseley, 2020).

5. Textual Analysis

Only a handful of selected COVID-19 updates were translated, and different Australian states seem to have adopted their own strategies to disseminate public health information in multiple languages.

The Australian Government Department of Health and Aged Care and the Queensland (QLD) Government have developed downloadable pamphlets of key information in "other" languages. The Government of Western Australia (WA) website shows a similar strategy and publishes downloadable translated documents on COVID-19 advice under four categories: Mandatory Contact Registers, COVID-19 Vaccination Program, Controlled Border Arrangement and WA Recovery Plan. However, the categories are not translated into an equal number of languages. As of September 9, 2021, information under Mandatory Contact Registers is in thirty-three languages; COVID-19 Vaccination Program, thirty languages; Controlled Border Arrangement, twenty-seven, and finally, WA Recovery Plan, in three languages only. In terms of Chinese languages, the website provides information on Mandatory Contact Registers and COVID-19 Vaccination Program in both Chinese (simplified) and Chinese (traditional), but Controlled Border Arrangement and WA Recovery Plan are in Chinese (simplified) only.

The New South Wales (NSW) Government website provides up-to-date information on the developing situation and the changing restrictions. The website boasts offering COVID-19 information in sixty languages other than English. The option of choosing different languages, however, comes with the disclaimer: "Our website uses an automatic service to translate our content into different languages. These translations should be used as a guide only." The Australian Capital Territory (ACT) Government adopts a similar approach, boasting the option of accessing its COVID-19 webpage in languages other than English with a note beneath each language "powered by Google Translate."

The Coronavirus (COVID-19) Victoria website and the South Australia (SA) Health website are the only ones displaying a comprehensive range of COVID-19 information in multiple languages with no disclaimer of an automated translation service. Rather than arraying multilingual pamphlet-like PDFs of the summary of key information as do the Australian Government, WA, and QLD Government websites, the VIC and SA Government websites attempt to offer the same content in multiple languages as that in English. In the language selection menu, however, while the Victorian Government website uses standard Chinese terms 简体中文 [jian ti zhong wen] for Chinese (Simplified) and 繁體中文 [fan ti zhong wen] for Chinese (Traditional), the SA Health website has mistranslated the two languages into 中國傳統 [zhong guo chuan tong] (lit. China traditions) and 中国简化 [zhong guo jian hua] (lit. China simplify).

A textual analysis of the Chinese-language COVID-19 information across states demonstrates the following key issues: trust in government, translation errors, inconsistency in terminology, cultural discrepancies, and lack of inclusiveness.

5.1 Trust in Government

Our students' responses to the Chinese translations of COVID-19 information on the Victorian Government website indicate a cultural expectation of the Chinese version published by government departments, that is, the quality of the Chinese version symbolises the government's credibility to and attitude towards the Chinese communities. Our students automatically treat the Chinese version as official documents, expecting it to be formal and free of errors. Inconsistencies, ambiguity, and frustrating reading experiences reflect poorly on the government. Awkward expressions and erroneous translations result in a lack of trust in the government's ability to care and manage the health crisis. Many of our students ask why the Victorian government would use machine translation for such important messaging, which may put community well-being and people's trust in the government at stake. As discussed earlier, there is in fact no evidence of the Victorian government using machine translation and our students tend to associate poor quality of translation with machine translation.

The presentation of translated resources, therefore, is not just a matter of good or bad editing—it may affect the users' trust in government. On June 29, 2021 Queensland Premier, Annastacia Palaszczuk announced that parts of South East Queensland, Townsville, Magnetic Island and Palm Island would enter into a three-day lockdown. On the same day, the government made a Simplified Chinese version of the directive available on its website. Notwithstanding time restrictions and the importance of ensuring important public messages being released to the public, the translation—despite being labelled as being written in "Chinese Simplified"—contained several passages written in traditional script. On June 26, 2021, New South Wales Premier, Gladys Berejiklian announced a fourteen-day lockdown for greater Sydney. The Chinese language website generated by automated translation displayed completely nonsensical messages. As we accessed the website on July 7, 2021, the website in Simplified Chinese was incomprehensible to the extent that premier was translated into "Prime Minister" and the Blue Mountains became "mountains which are blue in colour." Although the next day the website became more comprehensible, numerous mistranslations brought by machine translation, such as premier to Prime Minister, are still evident on the NSW Government website, along with awkward and ungrammatical expressions.

5.2 Translation Errors

On government websites where machine translation is not admitted to be in use, translation errors are still common; some more obvious, some more subtle. On January 31, 2021, the Premier of Western Australia, Mark McGowan, announced that the Perth metropolitan area, Peel and South West regions would enter into a five-day lockdown effective until February 5, 2021. Along with their English website, the Western Australian government published *COVID-19 coronavirus: Information and advice in Chinese (Simplified)*.

There were instances where the translated lockdown guidelines had omitted large portions of important health information. For example, people were required to stay at home unless they needed to:

> leave to exercise, but only within a 5km radius of your home for one hour per day. You can exercise with a maximum of 4 other members of your household, as long as there's no

more than 2 adults (e.g. one adult with up to 4 children from the same house, 2 adults with up to 3 children from the same house) and masks must be worn. (Government of Western Australia, 2022)

The Chinese translation distorted the original meaning and omitted several important details:

出门锻炼, 但同行者只限一人, 只允许在所在社区内, 每天仅限一个小时且必须佩戴口罩。 [*chu men duan lian, dan tong xing zhe zhi xian yi ren, zhi yun xu zai suo zai she qu nei, mei tian jin xian yi ge xiao shi qie bi xu pei dai kou zhao.*]

(back translation: leave to exercise, but only with one other person and only within the community you are in for a maximum of one hour per day, and masks must be worn.)

Another common translation error relates to the term "household," which is mistranslated into "家人" [*jia ren*] (lit. family members) on the Victorian Government website. The Australian Bureau of Statistics defines a household "as one or more persons, at least one of whom is at least 15 years of age, usually resident in the same private dwelling" (Australian Bureau of Statistics, 2021). In the context of the Victorian Government highlighting "large family gatherings" as one of the main triggers of the second wave of COVID-19 (Burton, 2020), the term "household" simply means people living under the same roof, without having to be family members. However, in the Chinese language and culture, the term "家人" [*jia ren*] (family members) is associated with the concept of "kinship" and refers to one's family members (Kang and Liu, 2009) who are related by blood, marriage, or adoption, but may or may not live together. If a Chinese reader were to read the translation, they would mistakenly believe that they can visit family members living in other residences. This mistranslation could potentially result in a violation of the Victorian Government's COVID-19 public health directions.

5.3 Inconsistency in Terminology

Comparing the translations of key terms such as "physical distancing" and "social distancing" on government websites across different states, we have identified significant inconsistencies in the translations, which may lead to greater confusion amongst the target audience.

Since the outbreak of the pandemic, the term "physical distancing" has appeared continually in Australia's COVID-19 public health communications as a recommended way of slowing the spread of the virus. According to the Australian Government, "physical distancing" in public means people should keep 1.5 metres away from others wherever possible, avoid physical greetings, exercise extra care in use of public transport, stay away from crowds, avoid large public gatherings, adopt good hygiene practices and stay at home in case of any COVID-like symptoms (Australian Government Department of Health and Aged Care, 2020b). Here, we can see "physical distancing" in the COVID-19 context has rich connotations, and getting the message across to Chinese-speaking communities in Australia can be a challenge. After surveying government websites across different states we find that the term "physical distancing" is translated into seven versions: "肢体距离" [*zhi ti ju li*] (lit. limb distancing), "身体距离" [*shen ti ju li*] (lit. body distancing), "物理距离" [*wu li ju li*] (lit. physics distancing), "身体疏远" [*shen ti shu yuan*] (lit. body drifting apart), "身体上的距离" [*shen ti shang de ju li*] (lit. distance between body parts) and "保持距离" [*bao chi ju li*] (lit. keeping at a distance). On one page of the South Australian Government website alone, "physical distancing" is translated into three different versions: "物理距离" [*wu li ju li*] (lit. physics distancing), "身体上的距离" [*shen ti shang de ju li*] (lit. distance between body parts) and "身体疏远" [*shen ti shu yuan*] (lit. body drifting apart), bringing to light the serious issue of inconsistency in key COVID-19-related terms. As the direct back translation of each of the seven versions shows, some hardly make any sense (such as "physics distancing" and "distance between body parts"), let alone convey the important message of "social distancing," and some sound awkward and confusing (such as "body drifting apart").

On the government websites across different states, we find three translations of "social distancing": "社交距离" [*she jiao ju li*] (lit. distancing during social interaction), "社会距离" [*she hui ju li*] (lit. distance between societies), and "社会疏远" [*she hui shu yuan*] (lit. societal drifting apart), with the first—社交距离 [*she jiao ju li*] (lit. distancing during social interaction)—being the most frequently used version. As the direct back translation shows, the three terms contain different connotations and only "社交距离" [*she jiao ju li*] (lit. distancing during social interaction) is a plausible candidate; while "社会距离" [*she hui ju li*] (lit. distance between societies) implies social stratification, and "社会疏远" [*she hui shu yuan*] (lit. societal drifting apart) carries a connotation of alienating someone socially. Therefore, notwithstanding similarities in the meaning of these various terms, a lack of consistency creates additional risks for confusion and misunderstanding.

5.4 Cultural Discrepancies

There are cultural concepts and practices in common Australian society but absent in the Chinese language which pose special translation challenges. One of the challenges involves translation of the term "compassionate reasons," which appears frequently throughout COVID-19 public health communications for exemptions applied to public health orders. There are two versions. The WA Government website uses "人道主义所提的要求" [*ren dao zhu yi suo ti de yao qiu*] (lit. requests made from humanitarianism), a rather awkward expression and the Victorian Government has "同情的理由" [*tong qing de li you*] (lit. sympathetic reasons). Neither translation is comprehensible to the Chinese reader unfamiliar with the Australian context. Translating "compassionate" into "同情" [*tong qing*] (sympathy) is problematic for two reasons.

First, there is a distinction between "compassion" and "同情" [*tong qing*], or sympathy. "Compassion" often refers to "a sensitivity to suffering in self and others with a commitment to try to alleviate and prevent it" (Gilbert et al., 2017, p. 1). However, "同情" [*tong qing*] (sympathy) is typically used in Chinese to describe the feeling of resonance and/or pity and sorrow for someone else's misfortune. As such, the Chinese concept of "同情" [*tong qing*] (sympathy) refers to the emotion rather than an active moral obligation or inclination to help others, and is equivalent to the concept of "sympathy" in English. This distinction is crucial as it exemplifies the differences in expectations on group and individual behaviour expressed through the two words: "compassion" and "同情" [*tong qing*] (sympathy).

Second, the problem intensifies when combined with the phrase "同情的理由" [*tong qing de li you*] (lit. sympathetic reasons). The phrase "compassionate reasons" is readily understood by native English-speaking residents of Australia. In the context of travel restrictions under COVID-19, it involves caregiving, tending to close friends or loved ones, attending funerals, etc., and is commonly used in the media, employment contracts, as well as the legal system (McAdam, 2011). However, the phrase "同情的理由" [*tong qing de li you*] (lit. sympathetic reasons) not only sounds awkward and nebulous, but also may lead to a misunderstanding of the message to be reasons for showing sympathy. As the phrase "compassionate reasons" in its general sense is absent in the Chinese language, a carefully deliberated term plus a thorough explanation is needed to convey the meaning behind the concept.

Another difficult word is "community," which appears throughout COVID-19 public health communications. The Victorian Government website translates "community" into "社区" [*she qu*] in all instances. The sentence "if we all follow the rules, we can protect our family, friends, and the community" is rendered into "若我们都遵守规则，我们就可以保护自己的家人、朋友和社区" [*ruo wo men dou zun shou gui ze, wo men jiu ke yi bao hu zi ji de jia ren, peng you he she qu*]. Some of our students find the translation misleading and missing an important message of collective responsibility and communitarianism in fighting against COVID-19. According to the Collins Dictionary, "community" means "all the people who live in a particular area or place" and also goes beyond to encompass "a group of people who are similar in some way" and "friendship between different people or groups, and a sense of having something in common." In this sense, the English word "community" focuses on "commonality" (Li, 2017) and is close to the concept of "society." By comparison, the concept of "社区" [she qu], having evolved over time in China, has been associated with "strong geographical and administrative characteristics" and is restricted to referring to those who live in a particular administrative area (Li, 2017). Translating "community" into "社区" [she qu] in this instance runs the risk of inviting the Chinese reader to focus on their suburban area only while the sense of collective responsibility for a wider community is lost. A more society-oriented Chinese translation would be more appropriate, for example, "社群" [she qun].

The word "metropolitan" and associated culture-specific terms have geographical referencing, such as "metropolitan Melbourne" (also known as "Greater Melbourne"), and "Greater Sydney." The Victorian Government defines metropolitan Melbourne as "the geographical area that defines Melbourne as a city and the capital of the state of Victoria" (Live in Melbourne, n.d.). As the Victorian Government introduces different restrictions to metropolitan Melbourne and regional Victoria, it is essential that accurate messages on the restrictions are sent to people, including those with no or limited English who live in or outside metropolitan Melbourne. This is where translation comes into play. However, our students find that the direct translation of "metropolitan Melbourne" into "墨尔本大都会区" [mo er ben da du hui qu] (lit. Melbourne big capital meeting district) ineffective in sending an accurate message. "Metropolitan Melbourne" may be a vague term to many Australians whose first language is English, but the translation process may add another layer of communication problems and a lack of explanation of the term in Chinese makes it impossible for the Chinese reader to understand what areas the term covers. Various translations observed on the NSW Government website reveal the same issue: "Greater Sydney" into "大悉尼" [da xi ni] (lit. a big Sydney), "大悉尼地区" [da xi ni di qu] (lit. a big Sydney area), or "更大的悉尼" [geng da de xi ni] (lit. a bigger Sydney).

5.5 Lack of Inclusiveness

Translation can be a process for or against social inclusion, as can be seen in our lexical choice when dealing with sensitive words. Gender bias and discrimination have been recognised as a prevalent problem in machine translation (Warner, 2021), so it is no surprise that the NSW Government website, which uses automated translation, contains numerous discriminatory expressions. These translations may be technically correct but fail to factor in cultural sensitivities, including disability culture.

Take the word "disability" itself as an example. On the Victorian Government's website, "disability" is translated to "残障" [can zhang]. Consequently, related phrases such as "people with a disability" and "disability care" are translated into respectful terms such as "残障人士" [can zhang ren shi] and "残障护理" [can zhang *hu li*]. On the NSW government website, which uses automatic language translation, the term "disability" is translated to "残疾" [*can ji*] and "残障" [*can zhang*] interchangeably, with the former being the more prevalent. Not surprisingly, on the NSW government website, phrases such as "a child with a disability" is translated into "残疾儿童" [*can ji er tong*] and "disability inclusion" is translated into "残疾包容" [*can ji bao rong*]. Indeed, both "残疾" [*can ji*] and "残障" [*can zhang*] are currently in use to refer to "disability" in official documents in China, the former being a more common usage. However, scholars and human rights advocates within China have long been arguing against the use of the former and calling for a change in the legal terminology to the latter (Liu, 2019). The phrase "残疾" [*can ji*] is made up of "残" [*can*], which literally means "damaged or injured," and "疾" [*ji*], which literally means "illness or disease" and has a tendency to suggest genetic defects. In comparison, replacing the character "疾" [*ji*] with "障" [*zhang*] which literally means "barriers" or "obstacles," the phrase "残障" [*can zhang*] avoids the undue reference to disease or infirmity. Rather, it signifies a recognition of barriers facing people with a disability and communicates the need for support without labelling them as "people with an illness," hence reducing risks for compromised human dignity. As government websites resort to machine translation, there are limited opportunities for human intervention to create inclusive language much needed in a public health crisis.

6. Conclusion

A rapidly evolving pandemic with massive societal disruptions calls for coordinated efforts in effective communication, and poor translation has serious social ramifications in a multicultural society such as Australia. Based on our study findings we arrive at the following recommendations for government translation work.

First, it is important in a multicultural society to treat translation as a cultural practice rather than a matter of box ticking. The quality of translation is fundamental to effective government—translation is not a mere linguistic exercise; it is an integral part of government messaging and crisis control and should be treated as such. This requires a paradigmatic shift in the mindset of governance, and critical assessment of multilingual and translation policies.

Second, it is important to have organised translation as a coordinated response to the pandemic in order to maintain consistency in terminology and messaging to ensure that information is conveyed efficiently and effectively. The global pandemic has highlighted the importance of recognising linguistic diversity, embracing social inclusion through language, and safeguarding the health and well-being of society by providing accurate and efficient translated health advice.

Across borders, translation is vital to ensure that linguistic minorities receive timely and accurate health information. For example, Al-Ma'ani, Al-Ajmi, and Al-Ajmi (2020) looking at COVID-19 translation in Oman, argue that community translation is a "soft force" in the fight against COVID-19. In Oman, 41.5% of the total population are 'non-Omanis,' and as such Oman was quick to recognise the importance of providing translation to linguistic minorities (Al-Ma'ani, Al-Ajmi, and Al-Ajmi, 2020). Community translation finds itself in the vanguard of the government response to COVID-19 and can be found in all the channels of communication including social media platforms, radio stations, TV channels, and official websites (Al-Ma'ani, Al-Ajmi, and Al-Ajmi, 2020).

Numerous cultural discrepancies suggest that multicultural Australia does not have the linguistic capacity to discuss and understand Australia's complex legal and political systems, cultural values, and social services in multiple languages. There is a lack of standardisation and explanation of commonly used terms in multiple languages. Translation is not solely for times of crisis.

Lachlan Thomas-Walters is a lawyer admitted in New South Wales. He holds a Master of Translation from the University of Melbourne, a BA (International Relations) and Bachelor of Laws (LLB) from the University of Queensland, and studied advanced Chinese and Chinese Law at Chongqing University and Shanghai Jiao Tong University.

Suqin Qian is a PhD candidate at the Asia Institute, University of Melbourne. Suqin Qian's research examines Chinese communities' experiences with translated COVID-19 resources in Australia. She holds a Master of Translation and Transcultural Communication from the University of Adelaide and Master of Translation from Beijing Foreign Studies University.

Delia Lin is Associate Professor in Chinese Studies, Asia Institute, University of Melbourne. Delia Lin has taught Chinese/English translation for three decades. Her research focuses on discourse, ideology, and social governance in a changing China, with a special interest in the role that words play in shaping political ideas.

Notes

[1] The authors would like to thank Yang Wang for her assistance with part of the research and the class of Translation, Interpreting, Communication in semester 2, 2020 and semesters 1 and 2, 2021 for their evaluation of Chinese translations of COVID-19 health information.

References

Aldridge, Ashlee, Sandra Moon, and Anna Chisholm. 2021. "COVID-19 rules change again for cross-border communities, causing confusion." *ABC News*, June 7, 2021. https://www.abc.net.au/news/2021-06-07/border-restrictions-change-again/100194794.

Allman, Kate. 2020. "Police state or safety net?: How NSW entered a strange 'new normal.'" *LSJ: Law Society of NSW Journal* 66: 30–35.

Al-Ma'ani, Musallam, Abdullah Said Al-Ajmi, and Sara Ali Al-Ajmi. 2020. "Community translation in the Sultanate of Oman: "A soft force" in the fight against COVID-19." *Journal of Arts and Social Sciences [JASS]* 11, no. 1: 5–13. https://doi.org/10.24200/jass.vol11iss1pp5-13.

Amat, Francesc, Andreu Arenas, Albert Falcó-Gimeno, and Jordi Muñoz. 2020. "Pandemics meet democracy: Experimental evidence from the COVID-19 crisis in Spain." *SocArXiv*. April 6. https://doi.org/10.31235/osf.io/dkusw.

Australian Bureau of Statistics. 2017. "Census reveals a fast changing, culturally diverse nation." Accessed May 8, 2022. https://www.abs.gov.au/ausstats/abs@.nsf/lookup/media%20release3.

Australian Bureau of Statistics. 2021. "Census of Population and Housing: Census Dictionary." Australian Bureau of Statistics. Accessed May 10, 2022. https://www.abs.gov.au/census/guide-census-data/census-dictionary/2021/glossary/h.

Australian Government Department of Health and Aged Care. 2020a. "Australian Health Sector Emergency Response Plan for Novel Coronavirus (COVID-19)." Australian Government Department of Health and Aged Care. Accessed May 10, 2022. https://www.health.gov.au/resources/publications/australian-health-sector-emergency-response-plan-for-novel-coronavirus-covid-19.

Australian Government Department of Health and Aged Care. 2020b. "Physical Distancing for Coronavirus (COVID-19)." Australian Government Department of Health and Aged Care. Accessed May 10, 2022. https://www.health.gov.au/news/health-alerts/novel-coronavirus-2019-ncov-health-alert/how-to-protect-yourself-and-others-from-coronavirus-covid-19/physical-distancing-for-coronavirus-covid-19.

Bakir, Caner. 2020. "The Turkish state's responses to existential COVID-19 crisis." *Policy and Society* 39, no. 3: 424–441. https://doi.org/10.1080/14494035.2020.1783786.

Bamford, Matt. 2020. "Confusing COVID-19 rules, chaotic approach concerns Sydney hospitality sector." *ABC News*, June 25, 2020. https://www.abc.net.au/news/2020-06-26/confusing-covid-rules-concern-for-sydney-hospitality/12373178.

Banerjee, Bratati. 2020. "COVID-19 containment: Legal framework for regulatory approach." *Journal of Comprehensive Health* 8, no. 2: 66–73. https://doi.org/10.53553/JCH.v08i02.002

Benítez, María Alejandra, Carolina Velasco, Ana Rita Sequeira, Josefa Henriquez, Flavio M. Menezes, and Francesco Paolucci. 2020. "Responses to Covid-19 in five countries of Latin America." *Health Policy and Technology*, 9, no. 4: 525–559. https://doi.org/10.1016/j.hlpt.2020.08.014.

Boseley, Matilda. 2020. "'It's so arbitrary': Melbourne street split down the middle by Covid-19 lockdown." *The Guardian*, July 2, 2020. https://www.theguardian.com/australia-news/2020/jul/02/its-so-arbitrary-melbourne-street-split-down-the-middle-by-covid-19-lockdown.

Brown, Jennifer. 2020. "Coronavirus: Parliamentary consent for the lockdown in England." *Insight*, May 4, 2020. https://commonslibrary.parliament.uk/coronavirus-parliamentary-consent-for-the-lockdown-in-england/.

Burton, Tom. 2020. "Victoria drops 'zero new cases' target in push for Christmas return." *Financial Review*, Oct 27, 2020. https://www.afr.com/policy/health-and-education/victoria-drops-target-of-zero-new-cases-before-removing-restrictions-20201027-p568wv.

Canestrini, Nicola. 2020. "Covid-19 Italian emergency legislation and infection of the rule of law." *New Journal of European Criminal Law* 11, no. 2: 116–122. https://doi.org/10.1177/2032284420934669.

Capano, Giliberto. 2020. "Policy design and state capacity in the COVID-19 emergency in Italy: If you are not prepared for the (un) expected, you can be only what you already are." *Policy and Society* 39, no. 3: 326–344. https://doi.org/10.1080/14494035.2020.1783790.

Chabibi, Busrol, and Irfan Jamallullail. 2020. "Are government appeals on physical distancing during the Covid-19 pandemic effective? An analysis from law and public policy." *Journal of Law and Legal Reform* 1, no. 4: 549–562. https://doi.org/10.15294/jllr.v1i4.39890.

Chiplunkar, Gaurav, and Sabyasachi Das. 2021. "Political institutions and policy responses during a crisis." *Journal of Economic Behavior & Organization* 185: 647–670. https://doi.org/10.1016/j.jebo.2021.03.018.

Christensen, Tom, and Per Lægreid. 2020. "Balancing governance capacity and legitimacy: How the Norwegian government handled the COVID-19 crisis as a high performer." *Public Administration Review* 80, no. 5: 774–779. https://doi.org/10.1111/puar.13241.

Civitarese, Jamil. 2020. "Social distancing under epistemic distress." *SSRN* 3570298. https://doi.org/10.2139/ssrn.3570298.

Committee on the Elimination of Racial Discrimination. 2020. "Statement on the COVID-19 pandemic and its implications under the International Convention on the Elimination of All Forms of Racial Discrimination." Committee on the Elimination of Racial Discrimination. Accessed May 10, 2022. https://www.ohchr.org/EN/HRBodies/Pages/COVID-19-and-TreatyBodies.aspx.

de Bruijn, Anne Leonore, Yuval Feldman, Malouke Esra Kuiper, Megan Brownlee, Chris Reinders Folmer, Emmeke Barbara Kooistra, Elke Olthuis, Adam Fine, and Benjamin van Rooij. 2020. "Why did Israelis comply with COVID-19 Mitigation Measures during the initial first wave lockdown?" *SSRN* 3681964. https://doi.org/10.31234/osf.io/vm8x9.

Gilbert, Paul, Francisca Catarino, Cristiana Duarte, Marcela Matos, Russell Kolts, James Stubbs, Laura Ceresatto, Joana Duarte, José Pinto-Gouveia and Jaskaran Basran. 2017. "The development of compassionate engagement and action scales for self and others." *Journal of Compassionate Health Care* 4, no. 4: 1–24. http://doi.org/10.1186/s40639-017-0033-3.

Government of Western Australia. 2022. "Perth metro, Peel and South West to enter hard lockdown." Government of Western Australia. Accessed March 10, 2023. https://www.wa.gov.au/government/announcements/perth-metro-peel-and-south-west-enter-hard-lockdown.

Judicial Commission of New South Wales. 2021. "People from culturally and linguistically diverse backgrounds." Judicial Commission of New South Wales. Accessed August 8, 2021. https://www.judcom.nsw.gov.au/publications/benchbks/equality/section03.html.

Kang, Shiyong and Hairun Liu, eds. 2009. *Xiandai hanyu xinciyu cidian* [The Contemporary Chinese New Dictionary] 2nd ed. Shanghai: Shanghai Lexicographical Publishing House.

Li, Lu. 2017. "The Development of the Concept of *Shequ* in Contemporary China, 1988–2016." Master's thesis, The University of Adelaide.

Liu, Pu. 2019. "Canji ren VS canzhang ren—ke qidai de falu yongyu zhuanhuan" [Can Ji Ren VS Can Zhang Ren—an expected shift in legal language]. *Human Rights* 6. http://www.humanrights.cn/html/2020/zxyq_0701/52270.html.

Live in Melbourne. n.d. "Metropolitan Melbourne." Live in Melbourne. Accessed August 8, 2021. https://liveinmelbourne.vic.gov.au/discover/melbourne-victoria/metropolitan-melbourne.

McAdam, Jane. 2011. "From humanitarian discretion to complementary protection-reflections on the emergence of human rights-based refugee protection in Australia." *Australian International Law Journal* 18: 53–76.

Mclean, Holly, and Ben Huf. 2020. "Emergency powers, public health and COVID-19." Research Paper 2: 70. https://doi.org/10.25916/5f39e5bb7f37f.

Nekvapil, Emrys, Maya Narayan, and Stephanie Brenker. 2020. "COVID-19 and the Law of Australia." Last updated June 21, 2020. https://covid19-law.com.au/ch-1-overview.html.

Parliament of Australia. 2020. "COVID-19 Australian Government roles and responsibilities: An overview." Parliament of Australia. Accessed May 10, 2022.https://www.aph.gov.au/About_Parliament/ Parliamentary_Departments/Parliamentary_Library/pubs/rp/rp1920/COVID19AustralianGovernmentRoles#_Toc40791054.

Piekkari, Rebecca, Susanne Tietze, Jo Angouri, Renate Meyer, and Eero Vaara. 2021. "Can you speak Covid-19? Languages and social inequality in management studies." *Journal of Management Studies* 58, no. 2: 587–591. https://doi.org/10.1111/joms.12657.

Piller, Ingrid. 2014. "Linguistic diversity and social inclusion in Australia." *Australian Review of Applied Linguistics* 37, no. 3: 190–197. https://doi.org/10.1075/aral.37.3.001edi.

Piller, Ingrid, Jie Zhang, and Jia Li. 2020. "Linguistic diversity in a time of crisis: Language challenges of the COVID-19 pandemic." *Multilingua* 39, no. 5: 503–515. https://doi.org/10.1515/multi-2020-0136.

Schalley, Andrea C., Diana Guillemin, and Susana A. Eisenchlas. 2015. "Multilingualism and assimilationism in Australia's literacy-related educational policies." *International Journal of Multilingualism* 12, no. 2: 162–177.

Victorian Legislation. 2020. *Public Health and Wellbeing Act 2008.* https://content.legislation.vic.gov.au/ sites/default/files/2020-05/08-46aa043%20authorised.pdf.

Victorian Ombudsman. 2020. "Investigation into the detention and treatment of public housing residents arising from a COVID-19 'hard lockdown' in July 2020." December 17, 2020. https://www. ombudsman.vic.gov.au/our-impact/investigation-reports/investigation-into-the-detention-and-treatment-of-public-housing-residents-arising-from-a-covid-19-hard-lockdown-in-july-2020/.

Warner, Andrew. 2021. "Addressing the gender bias in machine translation." *MultiLingual,* August 7, 2021. https://multilingual.com/addressing-the-gender-bias-in-machine-translation/.

World Health Organization. 2020. *COVID-19 STRATEGY UPDATE.* https://www.who.int/docs/default-source/coronaviruse/covid-strategy-update-14april2020.pdf.

Appendix 1. Restricted Activity Directions in Victoria

	Public Direction	Came into Force	Repealed
1.	*Restricted Activity Directions*	March 30, 2020	April 7, 2020
2.	*Restricted Activity Directions (No.2)*	April 7, 2020	April 13, 2020
3.	*Restricted Activity Directions (No.3)*	April 13, 2020	April 17, 2020
4.	*Restricted Activity Directions (No.4)*	April 17, 2020	April 24, 2020
5.	*Restricted Activity Directions (No.5)*	April 24, 2020	May 11, 2020
6.	*Restricted Activity Directions (No.6)*	May 11, 2020	May 11, 2020
7.	*Restricted Activity Directions (No.7)*	May 11, 2020	May 25, 2020
8.	*Restricted Activity Directions (No.8)*	May 25, 2020	May 31, 2020
9.	*Restricted Activity Directions (No.9)*	May 31, 2020	June 21, 2020
10.	*Restricted Activity Directions (No.10)*	June 21, 2020	July 1, 2020
11.	*Restricted Activity Directions (No.11)*	July 1, 2020	July 8, 2020
12.	*Restricted Activity Directions (Restricted Postcodes)*	July 1, 2020	July 8, 2020
13.	*Restricted Activity Directions (Restricted Areas)*	July 8, 2020	July 19, 2020
14.	*Restricted Activity Directions (No.12)*	July 8, 2020	July 19, 2020
15.	*Restricted Activity Directions (Restricted Areas) (No.2)*	July 19, 2020	July 22, 2020
16.	*Restricted Activity Directions (No.13)*	July 19, 2020	July 22, 2020
17.	*Restricted Activity Directions (No.14)*	July 22, 2020	July 30, 2020
18.	*Restricted Activity Directions (Restricted Areas) (No.3)*	July 22, 2020	August 2, 2020
19.	*Restricted Activity Directions (No.15)*	July 30, 2020	August 5, 2020
20.	*Restricted Activity Directions (Restricted Areas) (No.4)*	TBP—Repealed before commencement	August 2, 2020
21.	*Restricted Activity Directions (No.16)*	August 2, 2020	August 5, 2020
22.	*Restricted Activity Directions (Restricted Areas) (No.5)*	August 2, 2020	August 5, 2020
23.	*Restricted Activity Directions (Non-Melbourne)*	August 5, 2020	August 13, 2020
24.	*Restricted Activity Directions (Restricted Areas) (No.6)*	August 5, 2020	August 13, 2020

	Public Direction	Came into Force	Repealed
25.	*Restricted Activity Directions (Non-Melbourne) (No.2)*	August 13, 2020	August 16, 2020
26.	*Restricted Activity Directions (Non-Melbourne) (No.3)*	August 16, 2020	September 13, 2020
27.	*Restricted Activity Directions (Non-Melbourne) (No.4)*	September 13, 2020	September 16, 2020
28.	*Restricted Activity Directions (Restricted Areas) (No.7)*	August 13, 2020	August 16, 2020
29.	*Restricted Activity Directions (Restricted Areas) (No.8)*	August 16, 2020	September 13, 2020
30.	*Restricted Activity Directions (Non-Melbourne) (No.5)*	September 16, 2020	September 27, 2020
31.	*Restricted Activity Directions (Non-Melbourne) (No.6)*	September 27, 2020	October 11, 2020
32.	*Restricted Activity Directions (Non-Melbourne) (No.7)*	October 11, 2020	October 18, 2020
33.	*Restricted Activity Directions (Non-Melbourne) (No.8)*	October 18, 2020	October 25, 2020
34.	*Restricted Activity Directions (Non-Melbourne) (No.9)*	October 25, 2020	October 27, 2020
35.	*Restricted Activity Directions (Restricted Areas) (No.9)*	September 13, 2020	September 27, 2020
36.	*Restricted Activity Directions (Restricted Areas) (No.10)*	September 27, 2020	October 4, 2020
37.	*Restricted Activity Directions (Restricted Areas) (No.11)*	October 4, 2020	October 11, 2020
38.	*Restricted Activity Directions (Restricted Areas) (No.12)*	October 11, 2020	October 18, 2020
39.	*Restricted Activity Directions (Restricted Areas) (No.13)*	October 18, 2020	October 26, 2020
40.	*Restricted Activity Directions (Non-Melbourne) (No.10)*	October 27, 2020	October 28, 2020
41.	*Restricted Activity Directions (Restricted Areas) (No.14)*	October 26, 2020	October 27, 2020
42.	*Restricted Activity Directions (Melbourne)*	October 27, 2020	November 8, 2020
43.	*Restricted Activity Directions (Non-Melbourne) (No.11)*	October 28, 2020	November 8, 2020

	Public Direction	Came into Force	Repealed
44.	*Restricted Activity Directions (Victoria)*	November 8, 2020	November 22, 2020
45.	*Restricted Activity Directions (Victoria) (No.2)*	November 22, 2020	December 6, 2020
46.	*Restricted Activity Directions (Victoria) (No.3)*	December 6, 2020	December 9, 2020
47.	*Restricted Activity Directions (Victoria) (No.4)*	December 9, 2020	January 3, 2021
48.	*Restricted Activity Directions (Victoria) (No.5)*	January 3, 2021	January 29, 2021
49.	*Restricted Activity Directions (Victoria) (No.6)*	January 29, 2021	February 12, 2021
50.	*Restricted Activity Directions (Victoria) (No.7)*	February 12, 2021	February 17, 2021
51.	*Restricted Activity Directions (Victoria) (No.8)*	February 17, 2021	February 26, 2021
52.	*Restricted Activity Directions (Victoria) (No.9)*	February 26, 2021	March 15, 2021
53.	*Restricted Activity Directions (Victoria) (No.10)*	March 15, 2021	March 26, 2021
54.	*Restricted Activity Directions (Victoria) (No.11)*	March 26, 2021	April 9, 2021
55.	*Restricted Activity Directions (Victoria) (No.12)*	April 9, 2021	April 23, 2021
56.	*Restricted Activity Directions (Victoria) (No.13)*	April 23, 2021	April 30, 2021
57.	*Restricted Activity Directions (Victoria) (No.14)*	April 30, 2021	May 7, 2021
58.	*Restricted Activity Directions (Victoria) (No.15)*	May 7, 2021	May 25, 2021
59.	*Restricted Activity Directions (Victoria) (No.16)*	May 25, 2021	May 27, 2021
60.	*Restricted Activity Directions (Victoria) (No.17)*	May 27, 2021	June 3, 2021
61.	*Restricted Activity Directions (Metropolitan Melbourne)*	June 3, 2021	June 10, 2021
62.	*Restricted Activity Directions (Regional Victoria)*	June 3, 2021	June 10, 2021

	Public Direction	Came into Force	Repealed
63.	*Restricted Activity Directions (Metropolitan Melbourne) (No.2)*	June 10, 2021	June 12, 2021
64.	*Restricted Activity Directions (Regional Victoria) (No.2)*	June 10, 2021	June 12, 2021
65.	*Restricted Activity Directions (Metropolitan Melbourne) (No.3)*	June 12, 2021	June 17, 2021
66.	*Restricted Activity Directions (Regional Victoria) (No.3)*	June 12, 2021	June 17, 2021
67.	*Restricted Activity Directions (Metropolitan Melbourne) (No.4)*	June 17, 2021	June 24, 2021
68.	*Restricted Activity Directions (Regional Victoria) (No.4)*	June 17, 2021	June 24, 2021
69.	*Restricted Activity Directions (Metropolitan Melbourne) (No.5)*	June 24, 2021	July 1, 2021
70.	*Restricted Activity Directions (Regional Victoria) (No.5)*	June 24, 2021	July 1, 2021
71.	*Restricted Activity Directions (Regional Victoria) (No.6)*	July 1, 2021	July 29, 2021
72.	*Restricted Activity Directions (Metropolitan Melbourne) (No.6)*	July 1, 2021	July 29, 2021

Complete List of Works Cited

Abdullah, Faiz Sathi. 2014. "Mass media discourse: A critical analysis research agenda." *Pertanika Journal of Social Science & Humanities* 22: 1–18.

Abtahian, Maya Ravindranath, Naomi Nagy, Katharina Pabst, and Vidhya Elango. 2022. "Disruptions due to COVID-19: Using mixed methods to identify factors influencing language maintenance and shift." *Linguistics Vanguard* 8, no. s3: 331–341. https://doi.org/10.1515/lingvan-2021-0057.

Act on Special Measures for Pandemic Influenza and New Infectious Diseases Preparedness and Response 2020. (Japan). Accessed July 10, 2021. https://japan.kantei.go.jp/98_abe/statement/202003/_00001.html.

Ahn, Saerom. 2018. "Mitie tamlonulo pon nongchonyuhakuy uymi kwusengkwa silchen" [Discursive practices of schooling in farm villages in media discourses: A critical discourse analysis of the documentary *A Rural School, Urban Children*]. *Hwankyeng Kyoyuk* 31, no. 3: 224–240.

Aldridge, Ashlee, Sandra Moon, and Anna Chisholm. 2021. "COVID-19 rules change again for cross-border communities, causing confusion." *ABC News*, June 7, 2021. https://www.abc.net.au/news/2021-06-07/border-restrictions-change-again/100194794.

Allman, Kate. 2020. "Police state or safety net?: How NSW entered a strange 'new normal.'" *LSJ: Law Society of NSW Journal* 66: 30–35.

Al-Ma'ani, Musallam, Abdullah Said Al-Ajmi, and Sara Ali Al-Ajmi. 2020. "Community translation in the Sultanate of Oman: "A soft force" in the fight against COVID-19." *Journal of Arts and Social Sciences [JASS]* 11, no. 1: 5–13. https://doi.org/10.24200/jass.vol11iss1pp5-13.

Alyaa Alhadjri. 2020. "Groups say gov't's fake news awareness alert 'unclear, confusing.'" *Malaysiakini*, April 11, 2020. https://www.malaysiakini.com/news/520068.

Alyaa Alhadjri. 2021. "Bukit Mertajam MP claims no guidelines to appeal RM10k fine." *Malaysiakini*, March 14, 2021. https://www.malaysiakini.com/news/566552.

Amancio, R. Diego, Maria das Graças Volpe Nunes, Osvaldo N Oliveira, T.A.S. Pardo, L. Antiqueira and Luciano da F. Costa. 2011. "Using metrics from complex networks to evaluate machine translation." *Physica A: Statistical Mechanics and Its Applications* 390, no. 1: 131–142.

Amat, Francesc, Andreu Arenas, Albert Falcó-Gimeno, and Jordi Muñoz. 2020. "Pandemics meet democracy: Experimental evidence from the COVID-19 crisis in Spain." *SocArXiv*. April 6. https://doi.org/10.31235/osf.io/dkusw.

Andersson, Marta. 2021. "The climate of climate change: Impoliteness as a hallmark of homophily in YouTube comment threads on Greta Thunberg's environmental activism." *Journal of Pragmatics* 178 (June): 93–107.

Apple Daily. 2020. "E! Zhongguoren chi bianfu yingpian baoguang." [Ew! Video of Chinese people eating bats exposed]. January 23, 2020. https://tw.appledaily.com/international/20200123/WAT7R-JS3ZOUCSWPGM3GCAUZS5I/.

Asahi Shimbun. 2020a. "Shingata haien, dema ni chuui. 'Tokyo gorin chūshi,' 'chishiritsu 15%.'" [New type of pneumonia, be aware of misinformation: "Tokyo Olympics cancelled," "Mortality rate 15%."] January 1, 2020.

Asahi Shimbun. 2020b. "Korona taiō, hyōkasuru sēijka wa: Ichii wa Yoshimura Osaka fuchiji, nii wa Koike Tokyo tochiji. Asahi Shimbun yoron chōsa"[Asahi Shinbun survey. Corona response: which politician is highly evaluated? Osaka Governor Yoshimura at the top, Tokyo Governor Koike the 2nd.] December 30, 2020.

Asahi Shimbun. 2020c. "Korona to sabetsu: Shakai no kōhai o fusegu tame." [Corona and discrimination: To avoid dilapidation of the society.] April 19, 2020.

Asahi Shimbun. 2021. "'5th wave' of COVID-19 cases feared in Tokyo and Osaka." July 17, 2021. https://www.asahi.com/ajw/articles/14397380.

Asgeirsson, Hrafn. 2015. "On the instrumental value of vagueness in the law." *Ethics* 125, no. 2: 425–448.

Astrowani.com. 2020. "COVID-19: PKPD dikuat kuasa di dua kawasan di Simpang Renggam" [COVID-19: EMCO enforced in two areas in Simpang Renggam]. March 26, 2020. https://www.astroawani.com/berita-malaysia/covid19-pkpd-dikuat-kuasa-di-dua-kawasan-di-simpang-renggam-235454.

Australian Bureau of Statistics. 2017. "Census reveals a fast changing, culturally diverse nation." Australian Bureau of Statistics. Accessed May 8, 2022. https://www.abs.gov.au/ausstats/abs@.nsf/lookup/media%20release3.

Australian Bureau of Statistics. 2021. "Census of Population and Housing: Census Dictionary." Australian Bureau of Statistics. Accessed May 10, 2022. https://www.abs.gov.au/census/guide-census-data/census-dictionary/2021/glossary/h.

Australian Government Department of Health and Aged Care. 2020a. "Australian Health Sector Emergency Response Plan for Novel Coronavirus (COVID-19)." Australian Government Department of Health and Aged Care. Accessed May 10, 2022. https://www.health.gov.au/resources/publications/australian-health-sector-emergency-response-plan-for-novel-coronavirus-covid-19.

Australian Government Department of Health and Aged Care. 2020b. "Physical distancing for coronavirus (COVID-19)." Australian Government Department of Health and Aged Care. Accessed May 10, 2022. https://www.health.gov.au/news/health-alerts/novel-coronavirus-2019-ncov-health-alert/how-to-protect-yourself-and-others-from-coronavirus-covid-19/physical-distancing-for-coronavirus-covid-19.

Aw, Nigel. 2020. "Padah tersilap langkah, jangkitan Covid-19 berisiko melambung [Wrong move, Covid-19 infection at risk of soaring]. " *Malaysiakini*, March 18, 2020. https://www.malaysiakini.com/news/515266.

Aziz Ahmad. 2020. "Letter: Tired and exhausted at home." *Malaysiakini*, April 3, 2020. https://www.malaysiakini.com/letters/518567.

Bai, Gogentuul Hongye. 2020. "Fighting COVID-19 with Mongolian fiddle stories." *Multilingua* 39, no. 5: 577–586.

Bakir, Caner. 2020. "The Turkish state's responses to existential COVID-19 crisis." *Policy and Society* 39, no. 3: 424–441. https://doi.org/10.1080/14494035.2020.1783786.

Bakken, Børge. 2000. *The Exemplary Society: Human Improvement, Social Control, and the Dangers of Modernity in China.* New York: Oxford University Press.

Bamford, Matt. 2020. "Confusing COVID-19 rules, chaotic approach concerns Sydney hospitality sector." *ABC News*, June 25, 2020. https://www.abc.net.au/news/2020-06-26/confusing-covid-rules-concern-for-sydney-hospitality/12373178.

Banerjee, Bratati. 2020. "COVID-19 containment: Legal framework for regulatory approach." *Journal of Comprehensive Health* 8, no. 2: 66–73. https://doi.org/10.53553/JCH.v08i02.002

Bassnett, Susan. 2003. *Translation Studies.* London: Routledge.

Batagelj, Borut, Peter Peer, Vitomir Štruc, and Simon Dobrišek. 2021. "How to correctly detect face-masks for COVID-19 from visual information?" *Applied Sciences* 11, no. 5: 2070. https://doi.org/10.3390/app11052070.

Bélanger, Danièle, Hye-Kyung Lee, and Hong-Zen Wang. 2010. "Ethnic diversity and statistics in East Asia: 'Foreign brides' surveys in Taiwan and South Korea." *Ethnic and Racial Studies* 33, no. 6: 1108–1130.

Benítez, María Alejandra, Carolina Velasco, Ana Rita Sequeira, Josefa Henriquez, Flavio M. Menezes, and Francesco Paolucci. 2020. "Responses to Covid-19 in five countries of Latin America." *Health Policy and Technology*, 9, no. 4: 525–559. https://doi.org/10.1016/j.hlpt.2020.08.014.

Bernama.com. 2020. "COVID-19: Public to inform police for interstates travel." March 17, 2020. https://www.bernama.com/en/news.php?id=1822162.

Bernama/Malaysiakini. 2020a. "Permohonan rentas negeri hanya untuk warga kandas di kampung [Cross-state applications only for residents stranded in their hometowns]." April 23, 2020. https://www.malaysiakini.com/news/522199.

Bernama/Malaysiakini. 2020b. "Recovery MCO: Take stern action against nightclubs, pubs – Ismail Sabri." September 14, 2020. https://www.malaysiakini.com/news/542619.

Bernama/Malaysiakini. 2020c. "Covid-19 vaccine safety: Transparency vital to avoid public confusion", December 1, 2020. https://www.malaysiakini.com/news/553282.

Bernama/Malaysiakini. 2021a. "Parliament postponed on legal grounds to aid fight against Covid-19 – Takiyuddin." March 3, 2021. https://www.malaysiakini.com/news/565158.

Bernama/Malaysiakini. 2021b. "Annuar's SOP violation case: Police to record statements from witnesses." February 18, 2021. https://www.malaysiakini.com/news/563393.

Bhatia, Manjit. 2020. "A voice of reason and reassurance in Covid-19 fight." *Malaysiakini*, April 17, 2020. https://www.malaysiakini.com/news/521057.

Bhatia, Vijay. 1993. *Analysing Genre: Language Use in Professional Settings*. London/New York: Longman.

Blommaert, Jan. 2005. *Discourse: A Critical Introduction*. Cambridge: Cambridge University Press.

Blommaert, Jan. 2010. *The Sociolinguistics of Globalization*. Cambridge: Cambridge University Press. doi:10.1017/CBO9780511845307

Blumczynski, Piotr, and Steven Wilson, eds. 2023. *The Languages of COVID-19: Translational and Multilingual Perspectives on Global Healthcare*. New York: Routledge.

Borneo Post. 2020. "New business hours 8am-8pm for premises selling essential items starting April 1 – Ismail Sabri." March 30, 2020. https://www.theborneopost.com/2020/03/30/mco-new-business-hours-8am-8pm-for-premises-selling-essential-items-starting-april-1-ismail-sabri/.

Borton, Hugh. 1970. *Japan's Modern Century: From Perry to 1970*. New York: Roland Press.

Boseley, Matilda. 2020. "'It's so arbitrary': Melbourne street split down the middle by Covid-19 lockdown." *The Guardian*, July 2, 2020. https://www.theguardian.com/australia-news/2020/jul/02/its-so-arbitrary-melbourne-street-split-down-the-middle-by-covid-19-lockdown.

Boykoff, Jules. 2014. *Activism and the Olympics: Dissent at the Games in Vancouver and London*. Rutgers University Press.

Boykoff, Jules. 2017. "Protest, activism, and the Olympic Games: An overview of key issues and iconic moments." *International Journal of the History of Sport* 34, no. 3/4: 162–183.

Boykoff, Jules, and Matthew Yasuoka. 2014. "Media coverage of the 2014 Winter Olympics in Sochi, Russia: Putin, politics, and Pussy Riot." *Olympika: The International Journal of Olympic Studies* 23: 27–55.

Brown, Jennifer. 2020. "Coronavirus: Parliamentary consent for the lockdown in England." *Insight*, May 4, 2020. https://commonslibrary.parliament.uk/coronavirus-parliamentary-consent-for-the-lockdown-in-england/.

Burton, Tom. 2020. "Victoria drops 'zero new cases' target in push for Christmas return." *Financial Review*, Oct 27, 2020. https://www.afr.com/policy/health-and-education/victoria-drops-target-of-zero-new-cases-before-removing-restrictions-20201027-p568wv.

Butler, Judith. 2009. *Frames of War: When is Life Grievable?* London: Verso.

Byun, Jongseok. 2021. "Female marriage-migrants as safety and health care instructors: 'Prevention of mental illness.'" *Siheung Journal*, March 10, 2021. http://www.shjn.co.kr/news/articleView. html?idxno=60913.

Cabani, Adnane, Karim Hammoudi, Halim Benhabiles, and Mahmoud Melkemi. 2021. "MaskedFace-Net – A dataset of correctly/incorrectly masked face images in the context of COVID-19" *Smart Health* 19: 100144. https://doi.org/10.1016/j.smhl.2020.100144.

Canestrini, Nicola. 2020. "Covid-19 Italian emergency legislation and infection of the rule of law." *New Journal of European Criminal Law* 11, no. 2: 116–122. https://doi.org/10.1177/2032284420934669.

Capano, Giliberto. 2020. "Policy design and state capacity in the COVID-19 emergency in Italy: If you are not prepared for the (un) expected, you can be only what you already are." *Policy and Society* 39, no. 3: 326–344. https://doi.org/10.1080/14494035.2020.1783790.

Carlson, Rebecca, and Hiroto Hatano. 2023. "Branding a pandemic response: The biopolitics of (marketing) infection control in Japan." *Sociolinguistics Studies* 16, no. 4: 485–503.

Central News Agency. 2020. "Yidali beibu da fengcheng dan fangyi nan leguan: 'Women chengle xin Wuhan.'" [Northern Italy is locked down but no room for optimism in epidemic prevention 'we are the new Wuhan']. March 9, 2020. https://www.cna.com.tw/news/firstnews/202003090170.aspx.

Centre for Human Rights Education and Training 2020. STOP! *Corona Sabetsu: Sabetsu o nakushite tadashii rikai o kyanpēn* [Corona discrimination campaign: Eliminate discrimination and promote a correct understanding]. Accessed 1 July, 2021. http://www.jinken.or.jp/archives/21491.

Chabibi, Busrol, and Irfan Jamallullail. 2020. "Are government appeals on physical distancing during the Covid-19 pandemic effective? An analysis from law and public policy." *Journal of Law and Legal Reform* 1, no. 4: 549–562. https://doi.org/10.15294/jllr.v1i4.39890.

Chang, Angela, Peter Johannes Schulz, Sheng Tsung Tu, and Matthew Tingchi Liu. 2020. "Communicative blame in online communication of the COVID-19 pandemic: Computational approach of stigmatizing cues and negative sentiment gauged with automated analytic techniques." *Journal of Medical Internet Research* 22, no. 11. https://doi.org/10.2196/21504.

Channel News Asia. 2021. "COVID-19: Malaysia's recovery movement control order extended again to Mar 31." January 21, 2021. https://www.channelnewsasia.com/news/asia/malaysia-covid-19-rm-co-extended-mar-31-restrictions-13877484.

Chen, Chun-Mei. 2020. "Public health messages about COVID-19 prevention in multilingual Taiwan." *Multilingua* 39, no. 5: 597–606. https://doi.org/10.1515/multi-2020-0092.

Chen, Hantang. 2020. "Feiyan kunjingxia de yigong jiaolv." [Migrant worker anxiety under pandemic dilemma]. *Duli Pinglun*. March 14, 2020. https://opinion.cw.com.tw/blog/profile/52/article/9182

Chen, Kuan-hsing. 2010. *Asia as Method: Toward Deimperialization.* Durham and London: Duke University Press.

Cheng, Isabelle Cheng. 2020. "We want productive workers, not fertile women." *Asia Pacific Viewpoint* 61, no. 3: 453–465.

Chesnut, Michael, Nathaniel Ming Curran, and Sungwoo Kim. 2023. "From garbage to COVID-19: Theorizing 'Multilingual Commanding Urgency' in the linguistic landscape." *Multilingua* 42 no. 1: 25–53.

Chiplunkar, Gaurav, and Sabyasachi Das. 2021. "Political institutions and policy responses during a crisis." *Journal of Economic Behavior & Organization* 185: 647–670. https://doi.org/10.1016/j.jebo.2021.03.018.

Chong, Lip Teck. 2021. MCO: Malaysia Cincai Order. Sinchew News.com, 10 May 2021. https://www.sinchew.com.my/content/content_2474989.html.

Christensen, Tom, and Per Lægreid. 2020. "Balancing governance capacity and legitimacy: How the Norwegian government handled the COVID-19 crisis as a high performer." *Public Administration Review* 80, no. 5: 774–779. https://doi.org/10.1111/puar.13241.

Chung, Angie. Y, Hyerim Jo, Ji-won Lee, and Fan Yang. 2021. "COVID-19 and the political framing of China, nationalism, and borders in the US and South Korean news media." *Sociological Perspectives* 64, no. 5: 747–764.

Chung, Siaw-Fong. 2011. "A Corpus-based study of SARS in English news reporting in Malaysia and in the United Kingdom." *International Review of Pragmatics* 3, no. 2: 270–293.

Civitarese, Jamil. 2020. "Social distancing under epistemic distress." *SSRN* 3570298. https://doi.org/10.2139/ssrn.3570298.

Collins, Sandra. 2011. "East Asian Olympic desires: Identity on the global stage in the 1964 Tokyo, 1988 Seoul and 2008 Beijing games." *International Journal of the History of Sport* 28, no. 16: 2240–2260.

Committee on the Elimination of Racial Discrimination. 2020. "Statement on the COVID-19 pandemic and its implications under the International Convention on the Elimination of All Forms of Racial Discrimination." Committee on the Elimination of Racial Discrimination. Accessed May 10, 2022. https://www.ohchr.org/EN/HRBodies/Pages/COVID-19-and-TreatyBodies.aspx.

Commonwealth Magazine. 2020. "Yu Tan Desai zuodui 'Meilianshe:' Meiguo liyong yiqing tisheng Taiwan guoji diwei." [The Associated Press stands against Tedros: United States uses the pandemic to enhance Taiwan's international status]. April 9, 2020. https://www.cw.com.tw/article/5099792.

Coupland, Nik. 2020. Normativity, language & Covid-19. *Working Papers in Urban Language & Literacies* no. 271.

Dada, Sara, Henry Charles Ashworth, Marlene Joannie Bewa, and Roopa Dhatt. 2021. "Words matter: Political and gender analysis of speeches made by heads of government during the COVID-19 pandemic." *BMJ Global Health* 6: e003910.

Daijirin. 2006. 3rd ed. Tokyo: Sanseido.

Dang, Hoang Linh. 2021. "Social media, fake news, and the COVID-19 pandemic: Sketching the case of Southeast Asia." *Austrian Journal of South-East Asian Studies* 14, no. 1: 37–57.

Davies, Bethan L. Michael Haugh and Andrew John Merrison, eds. 2013. *Situated Politeness*. London: Bloomsbury Academic.

de Bruijn, Anne Leonore, Yuval Feldman, Malouke Esra Kuiper, Megan Brownlee, Chris Reinders Folmer, Emmeke Barbara Kooistra, Elke Olthuis, Adam Fine, and Benjamin van Rooij. 2020. "Why did Israelis comply with COVID-19 mitigation measures during the initial first wave lockdown?" *SSRN* 3681964. https://doi.org/10.31234/osf.io/vm8x9.

de Kloet, Jeroen, and Jian Lin. 2020. "'We are doing better': Biopolitical nationalism and the COVID-19 virus in East Asia." *European Journal of Cultural Studies* 23, no. 4: 635–640.

De Rycker, Antoon, and Zuraidah Mohd Don. 2013. "Discourse in crisis, crisis in discourse." In *Discourse and Crisis: Critical Perspectives*, edited by Antoon De Rycker and Zuraidah Mohd Don, 3–65. Amsterdam: John Benjamins Publishing Company.

Deraniyagala, Sonali. 2021. "Review of The Plague Year." *New York Times*, June 7, 2021. https://www.nytimes.com/2021/06/07/books/review/lawrence-wright-the-plague-year.html.

Dollinger, Marc J. 1988. "Confucian ethics and Japanese management practices." *Journal of Business Ethics* 7, no. 8: 575–584. https://doi.org/10.1007/bf00382789.

Dong, Jie. 2021. "Language and globalization revisited: Life from the periphery in COVID-19." *International Journal of the Sociology of Language* 2021, no. 267-268: 105–110. https://doi.org/10.1515/ijsl-2020-0086.

Droubie, Paul. 2011. "Phoenix arisen: Japan as peaceful internationalist at the 1964 Tokyo Summer Olympics." *The International Journal of the History of Sport* 28, no. 16: 2309–2322.

Du Bois, John W. 2007. "The stance triangle." In *Stancetaking in Discourse Subjectivity, Evaluation, Interaction*, edited by Robert Englebretson, 139–182. Amsterdam: John Benjamins Publishing Company.

Dunder, Ivan, Sanja Seljan, and Marko Pavlovski. 2020. "Automatic machine translation of poetry and a low-resource language pair." *43rd International Convention on Information, Communication and Electronic Technology (MIPRO)*, 1034–1039.

Dunn, Cynthia Dickel. 2006. "Formulaic expressions, Chinese proverbs, and newspaper editorials: Exploring type and token interdiscursivity in Japanese wedding speeches." *Journal of Linguistic Anthropology* 16, no. 2: 153–172. https://doi.org/10.1525/jlin.2006.16.2.153.

Dunn, Cynthia Dickel. 2011. "Formal forms or verbal strategies? Politeness theory and Japanese business etiquette training." *Journal of Pragmatics* 43 no. 15: 3643–3654.

Dunn, Cynthia Dickel. 2013. "Speaking politely, kindly, and beautifully: Ideologies of politeness in Japanese business etiquette training." *Multilingua: Journal of Cross-Cultural and Interlanguage Communication* 32, no. 2: 225–245.

Dunn, Cynthia Dickel. 2018. "Bowing incorrectly: Aesthetic labor and expert knowledge in Japanese business etiquette training." In *Japanese at Work: Politeness, Power, and Personae in Japanese Workplace Discourse*, edited by Haruko Minegishi Cook and Janet S. Shibamoto-Smith, 15–36. Cham: Springer International Publishing.

Edwards, Louise. 2010. "Military celebrity in China: The evolution of 'Heroic and Model Servicemen.'" In *Celebrity in China*, edited by Louise Edwards and Elaine Jeffreys, 21–43. Hong Kong: Hong Kong University Press.

Eelen, Gino, 2001. *A Critique of Politeness Theories*. Manchester: St. Jerome.

Eggins, Susanne. 1994. *An Introduction to Systemic Functional Linguistics*. London: Pinter Publishers.

Elster, Jon. 1989. "Social norms and economic theory." *Journal of Economic Perspectives* 3, no. 4: 99–117. https://doi.org/10.1257/jep.3.4.99.

Endicott, Timothy. 2011. "Vagueness and law." In *Vagueness: A Guide*, edited by Giuseppina Ronzitti, 171–191. Logic, Epistemology and the Unit of Science 19.

Everington, Keoni. 2021. "21 migrant workers in Miaoli questioned by police for venturing out." *Taiwan News*. June 9, 2021. https://www.taiwannews.com.tw/en/news/4219019?fbclid=IwAR1J9xlZo-hgp3Et-vC5yyWi-rbI26hfK33fQSh9zSioqwJMTRWw6QtBZAQU.

Fa Abdul. 2020. "Makcik Kiah must be very disappointed." *Malaysiakini*, August 12, 2020. https://www.malaysiakini.com/columns/538366.

Faisal Asyraf. 2021. "Wrong to fine one-year old child for not wearing mask, chides minister." *Malaysiakini*, February 25, 2021. https://www.malaysiakini.com/news/564369.

Fox, Colm A. 2021. "Media in a time of crisis: Newspaper coverage of Covid-19 in East Asia." *Journalism Studies* 22, no. 13: 1853–1873.

Freeman, Caren. 2011. *Making and Faking Kinship: Marriage and Labor Migration between China and South Korea*. Ithaca, NY: Cornell University Press.

Friedersdorf, Conor. 2021. "Australia traded away too much liberty." *The Atlantic*, September 2, 2021. https://www.theatlantic.com/ideas/archive/2021/09/pandemic-australia-still-liberal-democracy/619940/.

Gallois, Cindy and Shuang Liu. 2021. "Power and the pandemic: a perspective from communication and social psychology." *Journal of Multicultural Discourses* 16, no.1: 20–26.

Ge, Zhaoguang. 2017. *Lishi Zhongguo de nei yu wai* [Nei and Wai in Historical China]. Hong Kong: Chinese University of Hong Kong Press.

Gentzler, Edwin. 2017. *Translation and Rewriting in the Age of Post-Translation Studies*. New York: Routledge.

Gilbert, Paul, Francisca Catarino, Cristiana Duarte, Marcela Matos, Russell Kolts, James Stubbs, Laura Ceresatto, Joana Duarte, José Pinto-Gouveia and Jaskaran Basran. 2017. "The development of compassionate engagement and action scales for self and others." *Journal of Compassionate Health Care* 4, no. 4: 1–24. http://doi.org/10.1186/s40639-017-0033-3.

Girginov, Vassil and Laura Hills. 2008. "A sustainable sports legacy: Creating a link between the London Olympics and sports participation." *The International Journal of the History of Sport* 25, no.14, 2091–2116, https://doi.org/10.1080/09523360802439015.

Giulianotti, Richard, Gary Armstrong, Gavin Hales, and Dick Hobbs. 2015. "Sport mega-events and public opposition: A sociological study of the London 2012 Olympics." Article. *Journal of Sport & Social Issues* 39 no. 2: 99–119.

Goffman, Erving. 1967. *Interaction Ritual.* New York: Pantheon.

Goffman, Erving. 1974. *Frame Analysis: An Essay on the Organization of Experience.* Boston: Northeastern University Press.

Gogen Yurai Jiten. [Gogen Yurai Dictionary]. n.d. Accessed September 19, 2021. https://gogen-yurai.jp/.

Government of Malaysia. 1976. *Third Malaysia Plan, 1976-80.* https://policy.asiapacificenergy.org/sites/default/files/3rd%20MP.pdf.

Government of Western Australia. 2022. "Perth metro, Peel and South West to enter hard lockdown." Government of Western Australia. Accessed March 10, 2023. https://www.wa.gov.au/government/announcements/perth-metro-peel-and-south-west-enter-hard-lockdown.

Green, Marybeth, and C. Lisa McNair. 2019. "Steamsational writing: An investigation into using robots to inspire children's narrative skills." In *Handbook of Research on Integrating Digital Technology With Literacy Pedagogies,* edited by Pamela M. Sullivan, Jessica L. Lantz and Brian A. Sullivan, 175–191. Hershey: IGI Global.

Gries, Peter Hays. 2007. "Narratives to live by: The century of humiliation and Chinese national identity today." In *China's Transformations: The Stories Beyond the Headlines,* edited by Lionel M. Jensen and Timothy B. Weston, 112–127. Lanham: Rowman & Littlefield.

Gu, Yueguo. 1990. "Politeness phenomena in Modern Chinese." *Journal of Pragmatics* 14, no. 2: 237–257. https://doi.org/10.1016/0378-2166(90)90082-0.

Halliday, Michael. A. K. 1985. *An Introduction to Functional Grammar.* London: Edward Arnold.

Han, Peijie. 2017. "Quxiao yigong sannian xu chujing yiri yu shilian yigong renshu zhang zhi guanlianxing." [The connection between cancellation of need for migrant workers to leave the country at least one day in every three years and increase in numbers of missing workers]. *National Immigration Agency.* https://www.immigration.gov.tw/media/5988/%E5%8F%96%E6%B6%88%E7%A7%BB%E5%B7%A5%E4%B8%89%E5%B9%B4%E9%A0%88%E5%87%BA%E5%A2%83%E4%B8%80%E6%97%A5%E8%88%87%E5%A4%B1%E8%81%AF%E7%A7%BB%E5%B7%A5%E4%BA%BA%E6%95%B8%E6%88%90%E9%95%B7%E4%B9%8B%E9%97%9C%E8%81%AF%E6%80%A7.pdf.

Hassan, Hany, Anthony Aue, Chang Chen, Vishal Chowdhary, Jonathan Clark, Christian Federmann, Xuedong Huang et al. 2018. *Achieving Human Parity on Automatic Chinese to English News Translation.* Accessed June 18, 2021. http://arxiv.org/abs/1803.05567.

Haugh, Michael. 2013. "Im/politeness, social practice and the participation order." *Journal of Pragmatics* 58: 52–72.

He, Guanghua, Changyu Li, and Yuanzhou Cheng. 2020. "Wo shi dangyuan, wo xian shang!" [I am a Party member, I will go first!]. *People's Daily,* February 1.

He, Guanghua, Changyu Li, Yuanzhou Cheng, and Haotian Fan. 2020a. "Di-yi dao fangxian, shouzhu!" [First line of defence, stand strong!]. *People's Daily,* February 5.

He, Guanghua, Doudou Tian, Yuanzhou Cheng, and Shaotie Shen. 2020b. "Zhijing! Nixing de "baiyi zhanshi!" [We salute the 'soldiers in white' going against the current!]. *People's Daily,* February 2, 2020.

Heinrichs, Danielle H., Michael M. Kretzer, and Emily E. Davis. 2022. "Mapping the online language ecology of multilingual COVID-19 public health information in Australia." *European Journal of Language Policy* 14, no. 2: 133–162.

Helmbrecht, Johannes. 2002. "Grammar and function of *we*." In *Us and Others: Social Identities across Languages, Discourses and Cultures*, edited by Anna Duszak, 31–49. Amsterdam: John Benjamins.

Henley, Jon, and Caelainn Barr. 2020. "Global survey shows widespread disapproval of covid response." *The Guardian*, October 27, 2020. https://www.theguardian.com/world/2020/oct/27/global-survey-shows-widespread-disapproval-of-covid-response.

Ho, Ming-sho. 2020. "Watchdogs and Partners: Taiwan's civil society organizations." *Carnegie Europe*. December 7, 2020. https://carnegieeurope.eu/2020/12/07/watchdogs-and-partners-taiwan-s-civil-society-organizations-pub-83140?fbclid=IwAR0mkzQ6HQ7iJCWDaFBjvEqn5NhSF7WfBokfys2lkI5UlqlQjz7PlwqtFb4.

Hoang, Lan Anh. 2017. "Governmentality in Asian migration regimes: The case of labour migration from Vietnam to Taiwan." *Population, Space and Place* 23, no. 3: 1–12. https://www.mirrormedia.mg/story/20200512edi023/.

Hofstede, Geert. 1991. *Organization and Culture: Software of the Mind*. New York: McGraw-Hill.

Holthus, Barbara G., Isaac Gagné, Wolfram Manzenreiter, and Franz Waldenberger, eds. 2020. *Japan through the Lens of the Tokyo Olympics*. New York: Routledge.

Hong, Jinshan, Rachel Chang, and Kevin Varley. 2021. *The Covid Resilience Ranking: The Best and Worst Places to Be as Variants Outrace Vaccinations*. https://www.bloomberg.com/graphics/covid-resilience-ranking/.

Hong, Yihua, Changzoo Song, and Julie Park. 2013. "Korean, Chinese, or what? Identity transformations of Chosonjok (Korean Chinese) migrant brides in South Korea." *Asian Ethnicity* 14, no. 1: 29–51.

House, Juliane. 1977/1981. *A Model for Translation Quality Assessment*. Tübingen: G. Narr.

House, Juliane. 1997. *Translation Quality Assessment: a Model Revisited*. Tübingen: G. Narr.

House, Juliane. 2001. Translation Quality Assessment: Linguistic Description Versus Social Evaluation. *Meta* 46, no. 2: 243–257.

House, Juliane. 2009. *Translation*. Oxford: Oxford University Press.

House, Juliane. 2015. *Translation Quality Assessment: Past and Present*. London: Routledge.

Hubbard, Phil and Eleanor Wilkinson 2015. "Welcoming the world? Hospitality, homonationalism, and the London 2012 Olympics." *Antipode* 47, no. 3: 598–615.

Hwang, Kyongah. 2017. "Pantamwunhwa tamlonuy pwusangkwa enlonuy cayhyen = <cosenilpo>wa <hankyeleysinmwun>uy pantamwunhwa kwanlyen kisaey tayhan theyksuthupwunsekul cwungsimulo" [The paradox of multiculturalism reflected in media discourses: Representation of anti-multicultural sentiments]. *Mitie, Ceynte & Mwunhwa* 32, no. 4: 143–189.

Ibrahim Ali. 2020. "SURAT | Buat SOP biarlah masuk akal [Make an SOP that makes sense]." *Malaysiakini*, November 25, 2020. https://www.malaysiakini.com/letters/552515.

Iedema, Rick. 2001. "Resemiotization." *Semiotica* 137, no. 1: 23–39.

Iedema, Rick. 2003. "Multimodality, resemiotization: Extending the analysis of discourse as multi-semiotic practice." *Visual Communication* 2, no. 1: 29–57.

Imperial College London. 2020. "COVID-19 behaviour tracker." https://www.imperial.ac.uk/global-health-innovation/what-we-do/our-response-to-covid-19/covid-19-behaviour-tracker.

Inglis, David, and Anna-Mari Almila. (2020). "Un-masking the mask: Developing the sociology of facial politics in pandemic times and after." *Società Mutamento Politica* 11, no. 21: 251–257. https://doi.org/10.13128/smp-11964.

Ishiyama, Osamu. 2019. *Diachrony of Personal Pronouns in Japanese: A Functional and Cross-Linguistic Perspective*. Amsterdam: John Benjamins Publishing Company.

Jackson, Sarah J., and Brooke Foucault Welles. 2015. "Hijacking #Mynypd: Social media dissent and networked counterpublics." *Journal of Communication* 65, no. 6: 932–952.

Jang, In Chull, and Lee Jin Choi. 2020. "Staying connected during COVID-19: The social and communicative role of an ethnic online community of Chinese international students in South Korea." *Multilingua* 39, no. 5: 541–552. https://doi.org/10.1515/multi-2020-0097.

Japanese Red Cross Society. 2020. "*Shingata coronauirusu no mittsu no kao o shirō!: Fu no supairaru o tachikiru tameni.*" [Get to know the three faces of the novel coronavirus: To break out of a negative spiral.] Accessed July 1, 2021. https://www.jrc.or.jp/saigai/news/200326_006124.html.

Jary, Mark. 1998. "Relevance theory and the communication of politeness." *Journal of Pragmatics* 30, no. 1: 1–19.

Jeffreys, Elaine and Xuezhong Su. 2016. "Governing through Lei Feng: A Mao-era role model in reform-era China." In *New Mentalities of Government in China*, edited by David Bray and Elaine Jeffreys, 30–55. Abingdon: Routledge.

Ji, Pan. 2020. "Masking morality in the making: How China's anti-epidemic promotional videos present facemask as a techno-moral mediator." *Social Semiotics* 33, no. 1: 232–239. https://doi.org/10.1080/10350330.2020.1810462.

Jiang, Mengying. 2021. "Translating against COVID-19 in the Chinese context: A multi-agent, multimedia and multilingual endeavor." In *COVID-19 Pandemic, Crisis Responses and the Changing World: Perspectives in Humanities and Social Sciences*, edited by Simon X.B. Zhao, Johnston H.C. Wong, Charles Lowe, Edoardo Monaco, and John Corbett, 229–241. Singapore: Springer.

Jiang, Xinghan. 2020. "Yaoyuan youru xinguanbingdu! Yiguo Tairen: Yidali dengyu Wuhan kong yanguoqishi." [Rumours spread like the virus! Taiwanese in Italy: To say Italy is like Wuhan is an exageration]. *Global News Monthly*. March 13, 2020. https://www.gvm.com.tw/article/71574.

Jin, Di, Zhijing Jin, Joey Tianyi Zhou, and Peter Szolovits. 2020. A Simple Baseline to Semi-Supervised Domain Adaptation for Machine Translation. Manuscript accessed on June 18, 2021. https://doi.org/10.48550/arXiv.2001.08140.

Joo, Jaewon. 2012. "The discursive construction of discrimination: The representation of ethnic diversity in the Korean public service broadcasting news." PhD diss., London School of Economics and Political Science.

Judicial Commission of New South Wales. 2021. "People from culturally and linguistically diverse backgrounds." Judicial Commission of New South Wales. Accessed August 8, 2021. https://www.judcom.nsw.gov.au/publications/benchbks/equality/section03.html.

Kádár, Dániel Z., and Michael Haugh. 2013. *Understanding Politeness.* Cambridge: Cambridge University Press. https://doi.org/10.1017/CBO9781139382717.

Kaneyasu, Michiko. 2019. "The family of Japanese no-wa cleft construction: A register-based analysis." *Lingua* 217: 1–23.

Kang, Shiyong and Hairun Liu, eds. 2009. *Xiandai hanyu xinciyu cidian* [The Contemporary Chinese New Dictionary] 2nd ed. Shanghai: Shanghai Lexicographical Publishing House.

Khan, Mahmud Hasan, and Moses Stephens Gunams Samuel. 2020. "Confusion as an ideological tool in Malaysian newspaper op-eds." *CROSSINGS* 11: 225–241.

Kim, Anna. 2016. "Welfare policies and budget allocation for migrants in South Korea." *Asian and Pacific Migration Journal* 25, no. 1: 85–96.

Kim, Chul Kyu. 2009. "Personal pronouns in English and Korean texts: A corpus-based study in terms of textual interaction." *Journal of Pragmatics* 41, no. 10: 2086–2099.

Kim, Haneul. 2020. "Interpretation Support Group for Multicultural Families: Responding to COVID-19 in Step with Icheon City." *Gyeonggi Sisa Today*, April 13, 2020. https://www.yitoday.com/news/articleView.html?idxno=76101.

Kim, Hyun Mee. 2011. "The emergence of the 'multicultural family' and genderized citizenship in South Korea." In *Contested Citizenship in East Asia: Developmental Politics, National Unity, and Globalization*, edited by Kyung-Sup Chang and Bryan S. Turner, 203–217. New York: Routledge.

Kim, Kil Young, Dong Hwa Kim, Bok Hee Kim, Suk Ja Seong, Hye Kyeong Jang, Yun Jeong Cha, et al. 2003. *Hankwuke hwayonglon* [Korean pragmatics]. Seoul: Sejong.

Kim, Minjeong. 2008. "Gendering marriage emigration and fragmented citizenship formation: 'Korean' wives, daughters-in-law, and mothers from the Philippines." PhD diss., State University of New York, Albany.

Kim, Minjeong. 2010. "Gender and international marriage migration." *Sociology Compass* 4, no. 9: 718–731.

Kim, Yi-Gyeong, and Mee Sook Yoo. 2019. "Mamchwung homyengey tayhan tamlon pwunsek: Kisa pwunsekul cwungsimulo" [Discourse analysis of the use of the term *mamchoong* ("mum-roach"): Focusing on newspaper articles]. *Global Creative Leader: Education & Learning* 9, no. 1: 43–63.

Kimura, Ryoko. 2021. *"Yoshimura Osaka fuchiji no kōhyōka to posutoturūsu jidai."* [Positive evaluation of Osaka Governor Yoshimura and the post-truth era.] *Ronza*. May 12, 2021. https://webronza.asahi.com/culture/articles/2021051100007.html?page=2.

Kress, Gunther R, and Theo van Leeuwen. 2021. *Reading Images: The Grammar of Visual Design.* 3rd ed. Milton: Taylor & Francis Group.

Krystallidou, Demi, and Sabine Braun. 2022. "Risk and crisis communication during COVID-19 in linguistically and culturally diverse communities: A scoping review of the available evidence." In *The Languages of COVID-19: Translational and Multilingual Perspectives on Global Healthcare*, edited by Piotr Blumczynski and Steven Wilson, 128–144. New York: Routledge.

Kuk, Yeong Hi, and Ha Rim Jang. 2011. "Mitietamlon sok mwunhwayuhyengey kwanhan yenkwu – kayincwuuy nonuylul cwungsimulo" [A study of cultural patterns in media discourse: Focusing on the concept of individualism]. *Hankwukcachihayngcenghakpo* 25, no. 2: 177–195.

Lample, Guillaume and Alexis Conneau. 2019. *Cross-lingual Language Model Pretraining.* Accessed June 18, 2021. https://doi.org/10.48550/arXiv.1901.07291.

Latiff, Rozanna. 2020. "Malaysian leaders draw flak after post-election virus jump." Reuters, October 2, 2020. https://www.reuters.com/article/us-health-coronavirus-malaysia/malaysian-leaders-draw-flak-after-post-election-virus-jump-idUSKBN26N1SP.

Lee, Annabelle, and Hariz Mohd. 2020. "Dazed and confused: Covid-19 positive patients wait at home in limbo", December 30, 2020. https://www.malaysiakini.com/news/557037.

Lee, Boon Chye. 2020. "MP speaks | Face mask policy must be clear, without ambiguities." *Malaysiakini*, August 6, 2020. https://www.malaysiakini.com/news/537573.

Lee, Changsoo. 2019. "How are 'immigrant workers' represented in Korean news reporting?—A text mining approach to critical discourse analysis." *Digital Scholarship in the Humanities*, 34, no. 1: 82–99.

Lee, Han-Gyu. 2007. "Hankwuke taymyengsa 'wuli'" [A pragmatic and sociocultural approach to the so-called 1st person pronoun *wuli* in Korean]. *Tamhwawa Inchi* 14, no. 3: 155–178.

Lee, Hye-Kyung. 2014. "The role of multicultural families in South Korean immigration policy." In *Asian Women and Intimate Work*, edited by Emiko Ochiai and Kaoru Aoyama, 289–312. Leiden: Brill.

Lee, Hye-Kyung. 2015. "A corpus-pragmatic analysis of *Wuli*." *Tamhwawa Inchi* 22, no. 3: 59–78.

Lee, Hye-Kyung. 2020. "The use of the Korean first person possessive pronoun *Nay* vis-à-vis *Wuli*." *Language and Linguistics* 21, no. 1: 33–53.

Lee, Juheon, Sarah Cho, and Gowoon Jung. 2021. "Policy responses to COVID-19 and discrimination against foreign nationals in South Korea." *Critical Asian Studies*. https://doi.org/10.1080/14672715.2021.1897472.

Lee, Taewoong and Haein Lee. 2020. "Language barriers exacerbated by COVID-19 ... migrant women's struggle to learn Korean." *Hankook Ilbo.* May 13. https://www.hankookilbo.com/News/Read/202005251739393273.

Lee, Won-Pyo. 2005. "Sinmwun saseleyseuy inyem phyohyeney tayhan enehakcek pwunsek: 'kwukkapoanpep' phyeyciey tayhan noncaynguy kyengwu" [A linguistic analysis of ideologies in newspaper editorials: Focusing on the disputes about the abolition of the "National Security Laws"]. *Sahoyenehak* 13, no. 1: 191–227.

Li, Jia, Ping Xie, Bin Ai, and Lisheng Li. 2020. "Multilingual communication experiences of international students during the COVID-19 pandemic." *Multilingua* 39, no. 5: 529–539. https://doi.org/10.1515/multi-2020-0116.

Li, Keqiang. 2020. "Yao ba renmin qunzhong shengming anquan he shenti jiankang fang zai di-yi wei jianjue ezhi yiqing manyan shitou" [We must put the lives, safety and health of the masses first and resolutely curb the momentum of spread of the epidemic]. *People's Daily*, January 21, 2020.

Li, Lu. 2017. "The Development of the Concept of *Shequ* in Contemporary China, 1988–2016." Master's thesis, The University of Adelaide.

Liberty Times. 2020. "Dai kouzhao wufa xihu! Yilangren jie dangdi yiqing baofa guanjian yuanyin." [Can't breath with a mask on! Iranians reveal root of local outbreak]. March 17, 2020. https://ent.ltn.com.tw/news/breakingnews/3103147.

Liberty Times. 2020. "Wuhan feiyan: Taiwan fangyi weihe lingxian Riben? Xiangmin 8dian fenxi bei tuibao." [Wuhan Pneumonia – Why is Taiwan's epidemic prevention ahead of Japan's? Netizens' 8-point analysis tweeted widely]. February 16, 2020. https://news.ltn.com.tw/news/politics/breakingnews/3069564.

Lim, Donghoon. 2018. "Pragmatic effects of number and person in Korean pronominal system: Three uses of first person plural *Wuli.*" *Lingua* 204, (March): 1–15.

Lim, Ida. 2021. "In Malaysiakini decision, Federal Court acknowledges spotlight on free speech but reminds Malaysians to be polite online." *The Malay Mail*, February 19, 2021. https://www.malaymail.com/news/malaysia/2021/02/19/in-malaysiakini-decision-federal-court-acknowledges-spotlight-on-free-speec/1951082.

Lin, Vivi. 2020. "An Open Letter to Dr. Tedros." YouTube video. Accessed March 25, 2021. https://youtu.be/EKh6qiAGDfA.

Littlefield, Robert S. 2021. "Controlling the narrative: Mixed messages and presidential credibility." In *Communicating Science in Times of Crisis: COVID-19 Pandemic*, edited by H. Dan O'Hair and Mary John O'Hair, 358–374. Hoboken, NJ: John Wiley & Sons.

Liu, Shao-hua. 2020. "Feiyan yiqingxia tan jibing de mingming yu wuming." [On names and stigma in the pandemic]. *Duli Pinglun*. March 4, 2020. https://opinion.cw.com.tw/blog/profile/406/article/9150. For English translation, see https://www.readingthechinadream.com/liu-shao-hua-disease-names-and-stigma.html.

Liu, Kanglong and Andrew K. F. Cheung, eds. 2022. *Translation and Interpreting in the Age of COVID-19.* Singapore: Springer.

Liu, Pu. 2019. "Canji ren VS canzhang ren—ke qidai de falu yongyu zhuanhuan" [Can Ji Ren VS Can Zhang Ren—an expected shift in legal language]. *Human Rights 6.* http://www.humanrights.cn/html/2020/zxyq_0701/52270.html.

Liu, Xiao. 2020. "Yuanzhu quanqiu zhan 'yi' zhangxian daguo dandang (zhuanjia jiedu) " [Helping the whole world fight the pandemic demonstrates the responsibilities of a major power (an expert explains)]. *People's Daily*, March 30, 2020.

Live in Melbourne. n.d. "Metropolitan Melbourne." Live in Melbourne. Accessed August 8, 2021. https://liveinmelbourne.vic.gov.au/discover/melbourne-victoria/metropolitan-melbourne.

Loh, Jason. 2021. "Is the state of emergency justifiable at the end of the day? " *The Malay Mail*, January 15, 2021. https://www.malaymail.com/news/what-you-think/2021/01/15/is-the-state-of-emergency-justifiable-at-the-end-of-the-day-jason-loh/1940618.

Lommel, Arle, Aljoscha Burchardt, Maja Popović, Kim Harris, Eleftherios Avramidis, and Hans Uszkoreit. 2014. "Using a new analytic measure for the annotation and analysis of MT errors on real data." *Proceedings of the 17th Annual Conference of the European Association for Machine Translation (EAMT 2014)*. Accessed August 18, 2021. https://www.dfki.de/fileadmin/user_upload/import/7426_Lommel_el_al_2014_MQM.pdf.

Loo, Cindi. 2020. "CMCO ends June 9. Recovery MCO from June 10 to Aug 31." *The Sun Daily*, June 7, 2020. https://www.thesundaily.my/home/cmco-ends-june-9-recovery-mco-from-june-10-to-aug-31-updated-EM2538754

Low, Choon Chyuan. 2021. "MCO conundrum. 'He kept begging to move in. What were we to do?'" *Malaysiakini*, February 3, 2021. https://www.malaysiakini.com/news/561511.

M Fakrul Halim. 2021. "Physical SPM classes end on Feb 9, Maszlee urges minister to explain why." *Malaysiakini*, February 7, 2021. https://www.malaysiakini.com/news/562014.

Malay Mail. 2020. "Over 420,000 Malaysians sign petition objecting to CMCO which starts tomorrow." May 3, 2020. https://www.malaymail.com/news/malaysia/2020/05/03/over-420000-malaysians-sign-petition-objecting-to-cmco-which-starts-tomorro/1862546.

Malaysiakini. 2020a. " 'Confusing instructions' – Amanah Youth asks what PM and ministers doing." March 18, 2020. https://www.malaysiakini.com/news/515233.

Malaysiakini. 2020b. "Anwar urges gov't to provide complete info to lessen panic." March 18, 2020. https://www.malaysiakini.com/news/515216.

Malaysiakini. 2020c. "Yoursay: PM, we may have lost Covid-19 battle even before it started." March 20, 2020. https://www.malaysiakini.com/news/515618.

Malaysiakini. 2020d. "Only head of family allowed out for daily essentials, says senior minister." March 21, 2020. https://www.malaysiakini.com/news/515875.

Malaysiakini. 2020e. "Freight forwarders cry foul over contradictory instructions." 22March 2020. https://www.malaysiakini.com/news/516304.

Malaysiakini. 2020f. "Groups say gov't's fake news awareness alert 'unclear, confusing.'" April 11, 2020. https://www.malaysiakini.com/news/520068.

Malaysiakini. 2020g. "Putrajaya freezes MM2H applications, leaving agents confused." July 2, 2020. https://www.malaysiakini.com/news/532682.

Malaysiakini. 2020h. "Confused? Here's where and when to wear face masks." August 5, 2020. https://www.malaysiakini.com/news/537407.

Malaysiakini. 2020i. "DAP MPs criticise Putrajaya for confusion over work-from-home SOPs." October 22, 2020. https://www.malaysiakini.com/news/547563.

Malaysiakini. 2020j. "Ismail Sabri chuckles over confusion on 'work from home' SOPs." October 21, 2020. https://www.malaysiakini.com/news/547521.

Malaysiakini. 2020k. "Ismail sidesteps Yeoh's criticism, says people need to know actions taken." October 22, 2020. https://www.malaysiakini.com/letters/547656.

Malaysiakini. 2020l. "Families not allowed to circumvent 'two per household' rule in multiple vehicles." November 10, 2020. https://www.malaysiakini.com/news/550319.

Malaysiakini. 2020m. "Confusion over CMCO rules and other news you may have missed." November 11, 2020. https://www.malaysiakini.com/news/550368.

Malaysiakini. 2021a. "Singapore suspends travel bubble with Malaysia." January 30, 2021. https://www.malaysiakini.com/news/560996.

Malaysiakini. 2021b. "Emergency Ordinance grants Putrajaya sweeping powers against 'fake news.'" March 11, 2021. https://www.malaysiakini.com/news/566220.

Malaysiakini. 2021c. "It's back to nationwide MCO from May 12." May 10, 2021. https://www.malaysiakini.com/news/574152.

Malaysiakini. 2021d. "PM on SOP breach: Some got away due to lack of enforcers, but no double standards." May 23, 2021. https://www.malaysiakini.com/news/575848.

Malaysiakini. 2021e. "Nilai 3 is in S'gor' joke fails to tickle police's funny bone, probe initiated." May 24, 2021. https://www.malaysiakini.com/news/575864.

Malaysiakini. 2021f. "Rashid admits to attending durian feast recently, not last year." June 30, 2021. https://www.malaysiakini.com/news/581105.

Malaysiakini. 2021g. "Viral video of crammed MAEPS quarantine centre misleading – Nadma." January 9, 2021. https://www.malaysiakini.com/news/558284.

Malaysiakini. 2021h. "MCO 2.0 – what you can and can't do this time." January 13, 2021. https://www.malaysiakini.com/news/558704.

Malaysiakini. 2021i. "New MCO 2.0 rules: a guide to what's changed", January 30, 2021. https://www.malaysiakini.com/news/560983.

Malaysiakini. 2021j. "MMA blasts blame game over Covid-19 cases, wants apology." January 31, 2021. https://www.malaysiakini.com/news/561106.

Malaysiakini. 2021k. "MP: Instil greater awareness, not stiffer penalties to deal with Covid-19." February 1, 2021. https://www.malaysiakini.com/news/561270.

Malaysiakini. 2021l. "Confused and upset, politicians want new SOP for Chinese New Year." February 5, 2021. https://www.malaysiakini.com/news/561767.

Malaysiakini. 2021m. "Unity Ministry seeks review of SOP of Chinese New Year SOP celebrations." February 5, 2021. https://www.malaysiakini.com/news/561827.

Malaysiakini. 2021n. "Hua Zong denies taking part in talks with govt on CNY ruling." February 5, 2021. https://www.malaysiakini.com/news/561867.

Malaysiakini. 2021o. "Upcoming SPM exams need clear SOP early – educator." February 6, 2021. https://www.www.malaysiakini.com/news/561989.

Malaysiakini. 2021p. "Top cop concedes that enforcers find MCO SOPs confusing." February 8, 2021. https://www.malaysiakini.com/news/562045.

Malaysiakini. 2021q. "Daim: PN fails to instil confidence with confusing policies." February 15, 2021. https://www.malaysiakini.com/news/562971.

Malaysiakini. 2021r. "SOP violation: Minister says cops to decide, no need for DAP's judgment." February 16, 2021. https://www.malaysiakini.com/news/563153.

Malaysiakini. 2021s. "Interdistrict travel fine: Minister explains confusion." February 23, 2021. https://www.malaysiakini.com/news/564062.

Malaysiakini. 2021t. "MCO: Stiffer penalties and warrantless arrests under emergency rules." February 28, 2021. https://www.malaysiakini.com/news/564394.

Malaysiakini. 2021u. "RM10k fine fiasco." March 15, 2021. https://www.malaysiakini.com/newsletter/566586.

Malaysiakini. 2021v. "SURAT | Covid-19: Usah terhantuk baru tengadah [LETTER | Covid 19: Look up before getting hit]." January 2, 2021. https://www.malaysiakini.com/letters/557337.

Manabe, Noriko. 2016. *The Revolution Will Not Be Televised: Protest Music after Fukushima.* New York: Oxford University Press.

Manfredi-Sánchez, Juan-Luis, Adriana Amado-Suárez, and Silvio Waisbord. 2021. "Presidential Twitter in the face of Covid-19: Between populism and pop politics." *Comunicar* 66, no. 29, 83–94.

Markus, Hazel R., and Shinobu Kitayama. 1991. "Culture and the self: Implications for cognition, emotion, and motivation." *Psychological Review* 98, no. 2: 224–253. https://doi.org/10.1037/0033-295x.98.2.224.

Martin, J. R. 2004. "Mourning: How we get aligned." *Discourse & Society* 15, no. 2–3: 321–344. https://doi.org/10.1177/0957926504041022.

Mathayomchan, Boonyanit, Viriya Taecharungroj, and Walanchalee Wattanacharoensil. 2022. "Evolution of COVID-19 tweets about Southeast Asian countries: Topic modelling and sentiment analyses." *Place Branding and Public Diplomacy* 19: 317–334. https://doi.org/10.1057/s41254-022-00271-5.

Mazwin Nil Anis. 2020. "Family entertainment centres can reopen from July 15, says Ismail Sabri." *The Star*, July 10, 2020. https://www.thestar.com.my/news/nation/2020/07/10.

McAdam, Jane. 2011. "From humanitarian discretion to complementary protection-reflections on the emergence of human rights-based refugee protection in Australia." *Australian International Law Journal* 18: 53–76.

McGillivray, David, John Lauermann, and Daniel Turner. 2021. "Event bidding and new media activism." *Leisure Studies* 40, no. 1: 69–81.

Mclean, Holly, and Ben Huf. 2020. "Emergency powers, public health and COVID-19." Research Paper 2: 70. https://doi.org/10.25916/5f39e5bb7f37f.

Miller, Laura. 2017. "Japan's Trendy Word Grand Prix and Kanji of the Year: Commodified Language Forms in Multiple Contexts." In *Language and Materiality: Ethnographic and Theoretical Explorations*, edited by Jillian R. Cavanaugh and Shalini Shankar, 43–62. Cambridge: Cambridge University Press.

Mills, Sara, 2003. *Gender and Politeness*. New York: Cambridge University Press.

Ministry of Gender Equality and Family. 2018. *Cey3cha tamwunhwakacokcengchayk kiponkyeyhoyk (2018–2022)* [The third basic plan for multicultural family policy (2018–2022)]. Seoul, Korea: Ministry of Gender Equality and Family.

Ministry of Justice. n.d.. *"Korona sabetsu kaishō ni kansuru hōmushō no torikumi."* [Measures taken by the Ministry of Justice to eliminate corona discrimination.] Accessed July 10, 2021. http://www.moj.go.jp/JINKEN/stop_coronasabetsu.html.

Ministry of Labor. 2021. *109nian yigong guanli ji yunyong diaocha tongji jieguo 109* [Statistical Results of 2020 migrant worker management and utilization survey]. https://www.mol.gov.tw/media/90 36589/109%E5%B9%B4%E7%A7%BB%E5%B7%A5%E7%AE%A1%E7%90%86%E5%8F%8A%E9% 81%8B%E7%94%A8%E8%AA%BF%E6%9F%A5%E7%B5%B1%E8%A8%88%E7%B5%90%E6%9E %9C-%E5%90%AB%E5%9C%96%E8%A1%A8.pdf.

Ministry of Trade. 2021. *New Southbound Policy Implementation Plans.* https://newsouthboundpolicy.trade.gov.tw/English/PageDetail?pageID=49&nodeID=94.

Mirror Media. 2020. "Jingyou tu gangmeng: Zhi Wuhan feiyan? Yilangren tingxin pianfang yiqing jiaju." [Essential oils on the anus to treat Wuhan flu? Epidemic intensifies as Iranians follow folk remedies]. May 12, 2020. https://www.mirrormedia.mg/story/20200512edi023/.

Mohammad Firdaus Low Abdullah. 2020. "LETTER | Tackling the fake news pandemic." May 15, 2020. https://www.malaysiakini.com/letters/525769.

Molina, Pedro Santander. 2009. "Critical analysis of discourse and of the media: Challenges and shortcomings." *Critical Discourse Studies* 6, no. 3: 185–198.

Molnár, Anna, Lili Takács, and Éva Jakusné Harnos. 2020. "Securitization of the COVID-19 pandemic by metaphoric discourse during the State of Emergency in Hungary." *International Journal of Sociology and Social Policy* 40, no. 9/10: 1167–1182.

Mühlhäusler, Peter, and Ron Harré. 1990. *Pronouns and People.* Cambridge, MA: Blackwell.

Musolff, Andreas, Ruth Breeze, Kayo Kondo, and Sara Vilar-Lluch, eds. (2022). *Pandemic and Crisis Discourse: Communicating COVID-19 and Public Health Strategy.* London: Bloomsbury Academic.

Mutua, Makau. 2001. "Savages, victims, and saviors: The metaphor of human rights." *Harvard International Law Journal* 42, no. 1: 201–245.

Myers, Greg. 2010. "Stance-taking and public discussion in blogs." *Critical Discourse Studies* 7, no. 4: 263–275. https://doi.org/10.1080/17405904.2010.511832.

Myung, Minjun. 2020. "Co-participation of marriage-migrant women from Daegu in COVID-19 prevention." *Dong-a Ilbo*, June 30, 2020. https://www.donga.com/news/article/all/20200629/101741737/1?comm.

Na, Jinkyung, and Incheol Choi. 2009. "Culture and first-person pronouns." *Personality and Social Psychology Bulletin* 35, no. 11: 1492–1499.

Nadirah H. Rodzi. 2021. "Malaysia to impose MCO for two weeks in several states to curb Covid-19 cases – Muhyiddin." *The Straits Times*, January 11, 2021. https://www.straitstimes.com/asia/se-asia/malaysia-to-impose-mco-for-2-weeks-from-jan-13-in-several-states-to-curb-covid-19-cases.

Nakamura, Janice. 2022. COVID-19 signs in Tokyo and Kanagawa: Linguistic landscaping for whom? *Asia-Pacific Social Science Review* 22, no. 30: 80–94.

Nakayachi, Kazuya, Taku Ozaki, Yukihide Shibata, and Ryosuke Yokoi. 2020. "Why do Japanese people use masks against COVID-19, even though masks are unlikely to offer protection from infection?" *Frontiers in Psychology* 11. https://doi.org/10.3389/fpsyg.2020.01918.

Nanri, Keizo. 2005. "The conundrum of Japanese editorials: polarized, diversified and homogeneous." *Japanese Studies* 25, no. 2: 169–185.

Nekvapil, Emrys, Maya Narayan, and Stephanie Brenker. 2020. "COVID-19 and the Law of Australia." Last updated June 21, 2020. https://covid19-law.com.au/ch-1-overview.html.

New Straits Times. 2020a. "Covid-19: Movement Control Order imposed with only essential sectors operating." March 16, 2020.

New Straits Times. 2020b. "Certain businesses given green light to operate during MCO." April 10, 2020.

New Straits Times. 2020c. "NST Leader: RMCO extension the right move." August 29, 2020.

New Straits Times Online. 2020. "[LIVE] Special address by Prime Minister on the Recovery Movement Control Order (RMCO)." YouTube video. June 7, 2020. https://www.youtube.com/watch?v=btEfafQobeg.

NHK. n.d. "Kinkyū jitai sengen 1-kai-me no jōkyō" [First declaration of a state of emergency]. Accessed April 24, 2022 https://www3.nhk.or.jp/news/special/coronavirus/emergency/.

Nihon Dai Hyakka Zensho [Encyclopaedia of Japan]. 1994. Vol.18. 2nd ed. Tokyo: Shougakukan, 1994.

Nishimura, Yukiko. 2019. "Impoliteness." In *Routledge Handbook of Japanese Sociolinguistics*, edited by Patrick Heinrich and Yumiko Ohara, 264–278. London: Routledge

No 2020 Olympics Disaster OkotowaLink. 2020. *20 Reasons to Oppose the Tokyo Olympics.*

O'Hair, H. Dan and Mary John O'Hair. 2021. "Managing science communication in a pandemic." In *Communicating Science in Times of Crisis: COVID-19 Pandemic*, edited by H. Dan O'Hair and Mary John O'Hair, 3–14. Hoboken, NJ: John Wiley & Sons.

Oh, Steve. 2021. "Emergency puts democracy into an induced coma," *Malaysiakini*, January 29, 2021. https://www.malaysiakini.com/columns/560854.

Ohashi, Jun. 2008. "Linguistic rituals for thanking in Japanese: Balancing obligations." *Journal of Pragmatics* 40, no. 12: 2150–2174. https://doi.org/10.1016/j.pragma.2008.04.001.

Ohashi, Jun. 2021. "#MaskUp in Australia: How social norms in a pandemic are formed." *Melbourne Asia Review*. https://melbourneasiareview.edu.au/maskup-in-australia-how-social-norms-in-a-pandemic-are-formed.

Olympics.com. 2020. "Framework for the preparation of the Olympic and Paralympic Games following postponement." Accessed August 20, 2021. https://olympics.com/tokyo-2020/en/news/framework-for-the-preparation-of-the-olympic-and-paralympic-games-following-post.

Oostendorp, Marcelyn. 2018. "Extending resemiotisation: Time, space and body in discursive representation." *Social Semiotics* 28, no. 3: 297–314.

Ore, Adeshola. 2022. "Rights watchdog sees 1,445% spike in questions about Victorian government's powers during Covid." *The Guardian*, March 23, 2022. https://www.theguardian.com/australia-news/2022/mar/23/rights-watchdog-sees-1445-spike-in-questions-about-victorian-governments-powers-during-covid.

Papineni, Kishore, Salim Roukos, Todd Ward, and Wei-Jing Zhu. 2002. "BLEU: a method for automatic evaluation of machine translation." *Proceedings of the 40th Annual Meeting on Association for Computational Linguistics (ACL '02)*. Accessed August 16, 2021. https://doi.org/10.3115/1073083.1073135.

Park, Gil Ja. 2004. "Discourse analysis of school bullying videos." *Korean Journal of Youth Studies* 11, no. 1: 331–360.

Park, Harim. 2020. "Worse with COVID-19? 'Please help stop domestic violence in multicultural families.'" *News1*, June 19. 2020. https://www.news1.kr/articles/?3970163.

Park, Hyu-Yong. 2013. "Critical analysis of contrasting identities and styles of anti- and pro-multicultural discourses in Korea." *Sahoyenehak* 12, no. 3: 157–179.

Park, Mi Yung. 2017. "Resisting linguistic and ethnic marginalization: Voices of Southeast Asian marriage-migrant women in Korea." *Language and Intercultural Communication* 17, no. 2: 118–134.

Park, Mi Yung. 2019. "Challenges of maintaining the mother's language: Marriage-migrants and their mixed-heritage children in South Korea." *Language and Education* 33, no. 5: 431–444.

Park, Mi Yung. 2020. "'I want to learn Seoul speech!': Language ideologies and practices among marriage-migrants in South Korea." *International Journal of Bilingual Education and Bilingualism* 23, no. 2: 227–240.

Parliament of Australia. 2020. "COVID-19 Australian Government roles and responsibilities: An overview." Parliament of Australia. Accessed May 10, 2022.https://www.aph.gov.au/About_Parliament/Parliamentary_Departments/Parliamentary_Library/pubs/rp/rp1920/COVID19AustralianGovernmentRoles#_Toc40791054.

Pavlidou, Theodossia-Soula. 2014. "Constructing Collectivity with 'We': An introduction." In *Constructing Collectivity: "We" across Languages and Contexts*, edited by Theodossia-Soula Pavlidou, 1–22. Amsterdam: John Benjamins.

People's Daily. 2020a. "Meiguo guanyu xinguan feiyan yiqing de she Hua huangyan yu shishi zhenxiang" [America's lies concerning China about the novel coronavirus pneumonia epidemic, and the real truth]. May 10, 2020.

People's Daily. 2020b. "Chongfen fahui dangyuan ganbu xianfeng mofan zuoyong" [Bring into full play Party members' and cadres' pioneering and exemplary roles]. February 29, 2020.

People's Daily. 2020c. "Yiqing jiushi mingling Fangkong jiushi zeren" [The epidemic is an order, prevention and control is the responsibility]. January 26, 2020.

People's Daily. 2020d. "Jianding xinxin jianjue da ying yiqing fangkong zuji zhan" [Have steadfast confidence in resolutely winning the fight to prevent and control the epidemic]. January 26, 2020.

People's Daily. 2020e. "Wei daying yiqing fangkong zujizhan tigong youli baozhang" [Provide a strong guarantee to win the epidemic prevention and control blockade]. February 17, 2020.

People's Daily. 2020f. "Huijia" [Returning home]. April 7, 2020.

People's Daily Online. n.d. "Introduction to People's Daily." Accessed May 21, 2021. http://en.people.cn/90827/90828/index.html.

Petrovic, Sonja. 2020. "Tracing individual perceptions of media credibility in post-3.11 Japan." *The Asia-Pacific Journal: Japan Focus* 18, no. 10:3. https://apjjf.org/-Sonja-Petrovic/5397/article.pdf.

Pew Research Center. 2021. "A year of U.S. public opinion on the coronavirus pandemic." March 5, 2023. https://www.pewresearch.org/2021/03/05/a-year-of-u-s-public-opinion-on-the-coronavirus-pandemic/.

Piekkari, Rebecca, Susanne Tietze, Jo Angouri, Renate Meyer, and Eero Vaara. 2021. "Can you speak Covid-19? Languages and social inequality in management studies." *Journal of Management Studies* 58, no. 2: 587–591. https://doi.org/10.1111/joms.12657.

Piller, Ingrid. 2014. "Linguistic diversity and social inclusion in Australia." *Australian Review of Applied Linguistics* 37, no. 3: 190–197. https://doi.org/10.1075/aral.37.3.001edi.

Piller, Ingrid, Jie Zhang, and Jia Li. 2020. "Linguistic diversity in a time of crisis: Language challenges of the COVID-19 pandemic." *Multilingua* 39, no. 5: 503–515. https://doi.org/10.1515/multi-2020-0136.

Pizziconi, Barbara, 2006. "Politeness." In *Encyclopedia of Language & Linguistics*, edited by K. Brown, 679–684. 2nd ed., vol. 9. Oxford: Elsevier.

Pizziconi, Barbara. 2007. "The lexical mapping of politeness in British English and Japanese." *Journal of Politeness Research* 3, no. 2: 207–241.

PMO. 2020. Office of Prime Minister of Malaysia. Special Announcement of Emergency. https://www.pmo.gov.my/2021/01/teks-ucapan-pengumuman-khas-darurat/.

Popović, Maja. 2018. "Error classification and analysis for machine translation quality assessment." In *Translation Quality Assessment: from Principles to Practice*, edited by Joss Moorkens, Sheila Castilho, Federico Gaspari, and Stephen Doherty. Dordrecht: Springer International Publishing AG, 129–158.

Powell, Richard. 2020. *Language Choice in Postcolonial Law: Lessons from Malaysia's Bilingual System.* Singapore: Springer.

Raj, JS. 2020. "LETTER | Political ping pong amidst a pandemic." *Malaysiakini*, October 18, 2020. https://www.malaysiakini.com/letters/547004.

Ramieza Wahid. 2020. "Confusion leads Klang residents to police station for travel permission." *Malaysiakini*, October 8, 2020. https://www.malaysiakini.com/news/545806.

Ramieza Wahid. 2021a. "Ex-patient: Social stigma more painful than Covid-19." *Malaysiakini*, January 6, 2021. https://www.malaysiakini.com/news/557795.

Ramieza Wahid. 2021b. "Standardise MCO SOPs for all festivals, says Terengganu PKR chief." Malaysiakini, February 6, 2021. https://www.malaysiakini.com/news/561974.

Razak Ahmad, and Zakiah Koya. 2020. "Pakatan Harapan govt collapses." *The Star*, February 24, 2020. https://www.thestar.com.my/news/nation/2020/02/24/pakatan-harapan-govt-collapses.

Reconstruction Agency. n.d. "Recovery Olympics Portal Site." Accessed August 20, 2021. https://www.reconstruction.go.jp/2020portal/eng/.

Reiss, Katharina. 1989. "Text types, translation types and translation assessment." In *Readings in Translation Theory*, edited by Andrew Chesterman, 105–115. Helsinki: Oy Finn Lectura Ab.

Ren, Zhongping. 2020. "Fengyu wuzu xiang qian jin" [Neither wind nor rain will stop us from forging ahead]. *People's Daily*, March 26, 2020.

Reporters without Borders. 2021. *World Press Freedom Index.* https://rsf.org/en/ranking/2021.

Republic of China National Statistics. 2021. Accessed March 25, 2021. http://statdb.dgbas.gov.tw/.

Reuters Institute. 2019. *Digital News Report* 2019, 138-139. https://reutersinstitute.politics.ox.ac.uk/sites/default/files/inline-files/DNR_2019_FINAL.pdf.

Reuters/Malaysiakini. 2020. "Explainer: How does AstraZeneca's vaccine compare with Pfizer-BioNTech?" December 31, 2020. https://www.malaysiakini.com/news/557094.

Reyes Bernard, Natalie, Abdul Basit, Ernesta Sofija, Hai Phung, Jessica Lee, Shannon Rutherford, Bernadette Sebar, Neil Harris, Dung Phung, and Nicola Wiseman. 2021. "Analysis of crisis communication by the Prime Minister of Australia during the COVID-19 pandemic." *International Journal of Disaster Risk Reduction* 62, no. 1: 102375.

Rich, Motoko, and Hisako Ueno. 2020. "Japan's virus success has puzzled the world: Is its luck running out?" *The New York Times*, March 26, 2020. https://www.nytimes.com/2020/03/26/world/asia/japan-coronavirus.html – commentsContainer.

Roche, Gerald. 2020. "The Epidemiology of Sinophobia." *Made in China Journal*, January–April, 2020. https://madeinchinajournal.com/2020/02/17/the-epidemiology-of-sinophobia/.

Sakakibara, Ryota, and Hiroki Ozono. 2020. "Psychological research on the COVID-19 crisis in Japan: Focusing on infection preventive behaviors, future prospects, and information dissemination behaviors." *PsyArXiv* https://doi.org/10.31234/osf.io/635zk [Preprint].

Sakakibara, Ryota, and Hiroki Ozono. 2021. "Why do people wear a mask? A replication of previous studies and examination of two research questions in a Japanese sample." *The Japanese Journal of Psychology* 92, no. 5: 332–338. https://doi.org/10.4992/jjpsy.92.20323

Sakhiyya, Zulfa, Girindra Putri Dewi Saraswati, Zuhrul Anam, and Abdul Azis. 2022. "What's in a name? Crisis communication during the COVID-19 pandemic in multilingual Indonesia." *International Journal of Multilingualism*. https://doi.org/10.1080/14790718.2022.2127732.

Saldanha, Gabriela, and Sharon O'Brien. 2014. *Research Methodologies in Translation Studies*. Manchester: Routledge.

Sari, Ratna, Silvia Eka Putri, Herdi, and Budianto Hamuddin. 2018. "Bridging critical discourse analysis in media discourse studies." *Indonesian EFL Journal* 4, no. 2: 80–89.

Schalley, Andrea C., Diana Guillemin, and Susana A. Eisenchlas. 2015. "Multilingualism and assimilationism in Australia's literacy-related educational policies." *International Journal of Multilingualism* 12, no. 2: 162–177.

Schubert, Amelia L., Youngmin Lee, and Hyun-Uk Lee. 2015. "Reproducing hybridity in Korea: Conflicting interpretations of Korean culture by South Koreans and ethnic Korean Chinese marriage migrants." *Asian Journal of Women's Studies* 21, no. 3: 232–251.

Seargeant, Philip. 2011. "The symbolic meaning of visual English in the social landscape of Japan." In *English in Japan in the Era of Globalization*, edited by Philip Seargeant, 187–204. Basingstoke: Palgrave Macmillan.

Seljan, Sanja and Ivan Dunder. 2015a. "Automatic quality evaluation of machine-translated output in sociological-philosophical-spiritual domain." *10th Iberian Conference on Information Systems and Technologies (CISTI)*, 1–4.

Seljan, Sanja and Ivan Dunder. 2015b. "Machine translation and automatic evaluation of English/Russian-Croatian." *International Conference «Corpus Linguistics – 2015» (CORPORA 2015)*, 72–79.

Seljan, Sanja, Marko Tucaković, and Ivan Dunder. 2015. "Human evaluation of online machine translation services for English/Russian-Croatian." *3rd World Conference on Information Systems and Technologies (WorldCIST'15)*. Dordrecht: Springer International Publishing AG.

Sengupta, Papia. 2022. "Language, communication, and the COVID-19 pandemic: Criticality of multilingual education." *International Journal of Multilingualism*, 1–14, https://doi.org/10.1080/14790718.2021.2021918.

Sennrich, Rico, Barry Haddow, and Alexandra Birch. 2016. "Improving neural machine translation models with monolingual data." *Proceedings of the 54th Annual Meeting of the Association for Computational Linguistics (Volume 1: Long Papers)*. Berlin, Germany, 86–96.

Shen, Qi. 2020. "Commentary: Directions in language planning from the COVID-19 pandemic." *Multilingua* 39, no. 5: 625–629. https://doi.org/10.1515/multi-2020-0133.

Shiffman, Daniel. 2012. *The Nature of Code: Simulating Natural Systems with Processing.* Accessed June 19, 2021. http://natureofcode.com/.

Shin, Jaran. 2019. "The vortex of multiculturalism in South Korea: A critical discourse analysis of the characterization of 'multicultural children' in three newspapers." *Communication and Critical/ Cultural Studies* 16, no. 1: 61–81. https://doi.org/10.1080/14791420.2019.1590612.

Singelis, Theodore M. 1994. "The measurement of independent and interdependent self-construals." *Personality and Social Psychology Bulletin* 20, no. 5: 580–591. https://doi.org/10.1177/0146167294205014.

Smith, Aminda. 2020. "Of martyrs and maladies: Some thoughts on the coronavirus." *Positions Politics,* February 13, 2020. https://positionspolitics.org/aminda-smith-of-martyrs-and-maladies-some-thoughts-on-the-coronavirus/.

Sneller, Betsy. 2022. "COVID-era sociolinguistics: Introduction to the special issue." *Linguistics Vanguard* 8, no: s3: 303–306. https://doi.org/10.1515/lingvan-2021-0138.

Soames, Scott. 2012. "Vagueness and the law." In *The Routledge Companion to Philosophy of Law,* edited by Andrei Marmor, 95–108. New York: Routledge, 2012.

Sohn, Bong-Gi, and Mia Kang. 2021. "'We contribute to the development of South Korea': Bilingual womanhood and politics of bilingual policy in South Korea." *Multilingua* 40, no. 2: 175–198.

Song, Haseong. 2021. "Multicultural families unable to go home due to COVID-19: wait and hope." *Gyeonggi Multicultural Family News,* February 24, 2021. https://www.familynet.or.kr/download.do?uuid=ab088825-71a4-467b-b9eb-4c41607ac6bd.pdf.

Song, Heejin. 2013. "How international is EIL?: A critical discourse analysis of cultural representations in a Korean EFL education television program." *Critical Intersections in Education* 1, no. 2: 97–110.

Song, Jay. 2021. "The 'savage–victim–saviour' story grammar of the North Korean human rights industry." *Asian Studies Review* 45, no. 1: 48–66.

Song, Juyoung. 2019. "*Wuli* and stance in a Korean heritage language classroom: A language socialization perspective." *Linguistics and Education* 51, no. 3: 12–19.

Steentjes, Katharine, Tim Kurz, Manuela Barreto, and Thomas A. Morton. 2017. "The norms associated with climate change: Understanding social norms through acts of interpersonal activism." *Global Environmental Change* 43: 116–125. https://doi.org/10.1016/j.gloenvcha.2017.01.008.

Su, Sheng-Fang, and Yueh-Ying Han. 2020. "How Taiwan, a non-WHO member, takes actions in response to COVID-19." *Journal of Global Health* 10, no. 1: 1–5.

Suh, Kyung Hee, and Kyu-Hyun Kim. 2019. "Mitie tamhwauy piphancek tamhwapwunsek: tongnama icwumin kisalul cwungsimulo" [A critical discourse analysis of media discourse on Southeast Asian immigrants]. *Tamhwawa Inchi* 26, no. 3: 101–128.

Summers, Jennifer, Hao-Yuan Cheng, Hsien-Ho Lin, Lucy Telfar Barnard, Amanda Kvalsvig, Nick Wilson, and Michael G. Baker. 2020. "Potential lessons from the Taiwan and New Zealand health responses to the COVID-19 pandemic." *The Lancet Regional Health-Western Pacific* 2020: 100044.

Summerson Carr, E., and Michael Lepmert. 2016. *Scale: Discourse and Dimensions of Social Life.* Berkeley: University of California Press. https://doi.org/10.1515/9780520965430.

Super Daijirin. 2020. Tokyo: Sanseidō.

Surin, Jacqueline Ann. 2020. "Surviving the MCO and beyond." *Malaysiakini,* April 28, 2020. https://www.malaysiakini.com/columns/522872.

Suzuki, Takao. 1978. *Japanese and the Japanese: Words in Culture.* Tokyo: Kodansha. [Originally published in Japanese in 1973 as *Kotoba to Bunka,* Tokyo: Iwanami Shoten].

Taiwan International Workers Association. 2021. Accessed March 25, 2021. https://www.tiwa.org.tw/%e7%b5%84%e7%b9%94%e4%bb%8b%e7%b4%b9/tiwa%e7%b0%a1%e4%bb%8b/.

Tajfel, Henri, and John C. Turner. 1986. "The social identity theory of intergroup behavior." In *Psychology of Intergroup Relations,* edited by S. Worchel and W. Austin, 7–24. IL: Nelson-Hall.

Takigawa Christel-san kikoku: "Omotenashi" de Gorin shōchi [Ms Christel Takigawa arrives home: "Omotenashi" brings in the Olympic Bid]. *ANN News Channel* (You Tube), September 10, 2013. Accessed August 20, 2021. https://www.youtube.com/watch?v=PCFesHn_GRo.

Tan, KK, and Azmi Anshar. 2021. "COMMENT | Snap general election not needed to change govt." *Malaysiakini*, January 7, 2021. https://www.malaysiakini.com/columns/557976.

Tan, Nathaniel. 2020. "COMMENT | We need clarity, not confusion and red tape." *Malaysiakini*, November 14, 2020. https://www.malaysiakini.com/columns/550879.

Tan, Vincent. 2020. "Domestic travel bubbles approved in Malaysia as movement curbs lifted in four states." *Channel New Asia*, November 20, 2020. https://www.channelnewsasia.com/news/asia/malaysia-covid-19-domestic-travel-bubble-ismail-sabri-cmco-13601880.

The Japan Times. 2020. "Japan's low virus deaths reflect high 'cultural standards,' says Taro Aso". June 5, 2020. https://www.japantimes.co.jp/news/2020/06/05/national/japan-low-virus-deaths-high-cultural-standard-aso/.

The Star. 2021. "MCO violators face up to RM10,000 fine under amended Emergency Ordinance from March 11." February 25, 2021. https://www.thestar.com.my/news/nation/2021/02/25/rm10000-fine-for-mco-offences-under-new-emergency-ordinance-from-march-21.

The Tokyo Organising Committee of the Olympic and Paralympic Games. 2016. *Tokyo 2020 Action & Legacy Plan 2016: Participating in the Tokyo 2020 Games, Connecting with Tomorrow.*

Tian, Doudou, Yuanzhou Cheng, Haotian Fan, and Jun Wu. 2020. "Zhijing! Nixiang er xing de baiyi tianshi" [We salute the 'angels in white' going against the current!]. *People's Daily*, January 25, 2020.

Tokyo 2020 Website. 2013. "Christel Takigawa Joins Tokyo 2020 to Champion Cool Tokyo." 24 June 2013, Tokyo 2020 Website.

Tokyo Metropolitan Government. 2020. "STOP! Korona sabetsu." [Stop! Corona discrimination.] Accessed July 10, 2021. https://www.koho.metro.tokyo.lg.jp/2020/12/09.html.

Tombleson, Bridget, and Katharina Wolf. 2017. Rethinking the circuit of culture: How participatory culture has transformed cross-cultural communication. *Public Relations Review* 43 no. 1: 14–25. https://doi.org/10.1016/j.pubrev.2016.10.017.

Tong, Geraldine. 2020. "Is MCO necessary? Other countries didn't resort to lockdown, says Jomo." *Malaysiakini*, November 15, 2020. https://www.malaysiakini.com/news/550967.

Tovar, Johanna. 2023. "The role of language in place branding during the Covid-19 pandemic and post-lockdowns: An introduction." *Sociolinguistic Studies* 16, no. 4: 423–433. https://doi.org/10.1558/sols.23528.

Tsukimoro, Osamu. 2021. "With variants on the rise, Japan sticks to firm COVID-19 guidance." *The Japan Times*, July 6, 2021. https://www.japantimes.co.jp/news/2021/07/06/national/variants-japan-coronavirus-guidance/.

Turner, John C., Michael A. Hogg, Penelope J. Oakes, Stephen D. Reicher, and Margaret S. Wetherell. 1987. *Rediscovering the Social Group: A Self-Categorization Theory*. Oxford, UK: Blackwell.

U-can Neologism and Buzzword Award, 2013. Accessed August 20, 2021. https://www.jiyu.co.jp/singo/index.php?eid=00030.

van Dijk, Teun A. 1993a. "Principles of critical discourse analysis". *Discourse & Society* 4, no. 2: 249–283.

van Dijk, Teun A.1993b. *Elite Discourse and Racism*. Thousand Oaks: SAGE Publications.

van Dijk, Teun A. 1998. "Opinions and ideologies in the press". In *Approaches to Media Discourse*, edited by Allan Bell and Peter Garrett, 21–63. Oxford: Blackwell.

van Dijk, Teun A. 2006. "Discourse and manipulation". *Discourse & Society* 17, no. 3: 359–383.

Vaswani, Ashwin, Samy Bengio, Eugene Brevdo, Francois Chollet, Aidan N. Gomez, Stephan Gouws, Llion Jones, Łukasz Kaiser, Nal Kalchbrenner, Niki Parmar, Ryan Sepassi, Noam Shazeer, and

Jakob Uszkoreit. 2018. *Tensor2tensor for Neural Machine Translation*. Accessed August 18, 2021. https://arxiv.org/abs/1803.07416.

Vazquez, Marietta. 2020. "Calling COVID-19 the 'Wuhan Virus' or 'China Virus' is inaccurate and xenophobic." *Yale School of Medicine*, March 12, 2020. https://medicine.yale.edu/news-article/calling-covid-19-the-wuhan-virus-or-china-virus-is-inaccurate-and-xenophobic/.

Victorian Legislation. 2020. *Public Health and Wellbeing Act 2008*. https://content.legislation.vic.gov.au/sites/default/files/2020-05/08-46aa043%20authorised.pdf.

Victorian Ombudsman. 2020. "Investigation into the detention and treatment of public housing residents arising from a COVID-19 'hard lockdown' in July 2020." December 17, 2020. https://www.ombudsman.vic.gov.au/our-impact/investigation-reports/investigation-into-the-detention-and-treatment-of-public-housing-residents-arising-from-a-covid-19-hard-lockdown-in-july-2020/.

Vitorio, Raymund, and Paolo Niño Valdez. 2023. "The taming of the shrewd: Technologies of the self, emotions, and the rebranding of Philippine tourism." *Sociolinguistic Studies* 16, no. 4: 505–524. https://doi.org/10.1558/sols.23527.

Wang, Haiyang, Colin Sparks, and Yu Huang. 2018. "Measuring differences in the Chinese press: A study of People's Daily and Southern Metropolitan Daily." *Global Media and China* 3, no. 3: 125–140.

Wang, Hui. 2014. *Xiandai Zhongguo sixiang de xingqi* [The Rise of Modern Chinese Thought]. Beijing: Sanlian shudian.

Warner, Andrew. 2021. "Addressing the gender bias in machine translation." *MultiLingual*, August 7, 2021. https://multilingual.com/addressing-the-gender-bias-in-machine-translation/.

Watts, Richard J. 1992. "Linguistic politeness and politic verbal behaviour: Reconsidering claim for universality." In *Politeness in Language: Studies in its History, Theory and Practice*, edited by Richard Watts, Sachiko Ide, Konrad Ehlich, 43–69. Berlin: Mouton de Gruyter.

Watts, Richard J. 2003. *Politeness*. Key Topics in Sociolinguistics. Cambridge: Cambridge University Press. https://doi.org/10.1017/CBO9780511615184.

Welsh, Bridget. 2020. "COMMENT | The unsung role of state gov'ts in battling Covid." *Malaysiakini*, July 3, 2020. https://www.malaysiakini.com/columns/532836.

Wenger, Etienne.1998. *Communities of Practice: Learning, Meaning, and Identity*. New York: Cambridge University Press.

Wingfield-Hayes, Rupert. 2020. "Coronavirus: Japan's mysteriously low virus death rate." *BBC News*, July 4, 2020. https://www.bbc.com/news/world-asia-53188847.

World Health Organization. 2020. *COVID-19 STRATEGY UPDATE*. https://www.who.int/docs/default-source/coronaviruse/covid-strategy-update-14april2020.pdf.

World Health Organization. 2021. "Coronavirus disease (COVID-19) pandemic." https://www.who.int/emergencies/diseases/novel-coronavirus-2019.

World Health Organization. n.d. "COVID-19: Addressing social stigma and discrimination." World Health Organization. Accessed August 13, 2021. https://www.who.int/westernpacific/emergencies/covid-19/information/social-stigma-discrimination.

Wu, Jingru. 2021. "Fandui Miaolixian zhengfu xianzhi yigong waichu." [Oppose the Miaoli County Government Prohibiting Migrant Workers from Going Out] *Taiwan International Workers' Association*. June 10, 2021. https://www.tiwa.org.tw/%E3%80%90%E6%96%B0%E8%81%9E%E7%A8%BF%E3%80%91%E5%8F%8D%E5%B0%8D%E8%8B%97%E6%A0%97%E7%B8%A3%E6%94%BF%E5%BA%9C%E9%99%90%E5%88%B6%E7%A7%BB%E5%B7%A5%E5%A4%96%E5%87%BA-%E7%B7%9A%E4%B8%8A%E8%A8%98%E8%80%85/.

Xiao, Tingfang. 2020. "Taiwan cheng da heigong tiantang... wufa qiansong huiguo de shilian yigong." [Taiwan now paradise for illegal workers...Why do uncontactable migrant workers who can't be sent home roam the country and even increase their price?] *Taiwan United Daily News*, December 10, 2020. https://udn.com/news/story/6839/5081188.

Xie, Mengying. 2020. "'Guojia conglai mei ba tamen dangren kan!' 108ming yigong quezhen. Mintuan jie zhenzheng 'fangyi pokou.'" ['The country has never seen them as people!' 108 migrant workers test positive, reveal weak link in epidemic prevention chain]. *Storm Media*, December 10, 2020. https://www.storm.mg/article/3283645?page=3.

Xiong, Ying, Moonhee Cho, and Brandon Boatwright. 2019. "Hashtag activism and message frames among social movement organizations: Semantic network analysis and thematic analysis of Twitter during the #MeToo movement." *Public Relations Review* 45, no. 1: 10–23.

Yang, Guobin. 2016. "Narrative agency in hashtag activism: The case of #BlackLivesMatter." *Media and Communication* 4, no. 4: 13–17.

Yang Lai Fong, and Leong Wai Kit. 2016. "Different political beliefs and different frame building for an inter-religious conflict: A comparative analysis of The Star and Malaysiakini." *Global Media Journal*, 2016. https://www.globalmediajournal.com/open-access/different-political-beliefs-and-d.

Yi Rong Hoo, Billy. 2020. "Detention centres poised to form coronavirus clusters." *Malaysiakini*, April 23, 2020. https://www.malaysiakini.com/news/522111.

Yin, Jason Dean-Chen. 2021. "WHO, COVID-19, and Taiwan as the Ghost Island." *Global Public Health*, February 26, 2021. https://doi.org/10.1080/17441692.2021.1890184.

Yomiuri Shimbun. 2020a. *"Kikokusha taiō seifu kuryo. Bukan daiichibin."* [Government facing difficulties with returnees. First repatriation flight from Wuhan.] January 30, 2020.

Yomiuri Shimbun. 2020b. *"Korona kajō hannō: Henken wa shakai fuan shika umanai."* [Overreaction to corona: Prejudice only causes social unrest.] April 23, 2020.

Yoon, Jae Hak. 2003. "Tanswucek yongpepuy wuli" [The singular usage of *wuli*]. *Enewa Cengpo* 7, no. 2: 1–30.

Zappavigna, Michele. 2015. "Searchable talk: The linguistic functions of hashtags." *Social Semiotics* 25. no. 3: 274–291.

Zhang, Jie, and Yuqin Wu. 2020. "Providing multilingual logistics communication in COVID-19 disaster relief." *Multilingua* 39, no. 5: 517–528. https://doi.org/10.1515/multi-2020-0110.

Zhang, Leticia-Tian and Sumin Zhao. 2020. "Diaspora micro-influencers and COVID-19 communication on social media: The case of Chinese-speaking YouTube vloggers." *Multilingua* 39, no. 5, 553–563. https://doi.org/10.1515/multi-2020-0099.

Zhao, Simon X.B., Johnston H.C. Wong, Charles Lowe, Edoardo Monaco, and John Corbett, eds. 2021. *COVID-19 Pandemic, Crisis Responses and the Changing World: Perspectives in Humanities and Social Sciences.* Singapore: Springer.

Zhao, Suisheng. 1998. "A state-led nationalism: The patriotic education campaign in Post-Tiananmen China." *Communist and Post-Communist Studies* 31, no. 3: 287–302.

Zheng, Yongyan. 2020. "Mobilizing foreign language students for multilingual crisis translation in Shanghai." *Multilingua* 39, no. 5: 587–595. https://doi.org/10.1515/multi-2020-0095.

Zhong, Sheng. 2020a. "Zhui ze suopei naoju shi wenming zhi chi" [Farcically claiming damages is a disgrace to civility]. *People's Daily*, May 3, 2020.

Zhong, Sheng. 2020b. "'Shuai guo' qineng zhengjiu shengming" [How could 'passing the buck' save lives?]. *People's Daily*, May 2.

Zhong, Sheng. 2020c. "Moshi 'shengming zhishang' he tan renquan" [How can you talk of human rights when you ignore the 'sanctity of life'?]. *People's Daily*, May 4, 2020.

Zhong, Sheng. 2020d. "Konghan 'airen ru ji' shize zisi lengxue" [Prattling on about 'loving others as you love yourself,' but in actuality selfish and cold-blooded]. *People's Daily*, May 6, 2020.

Zhong, Sheng. 2020e. "Wuming hua shi weixian de 'zhengzhi bingdu'" [Stigmatisation is a dangerous "political virus"]. *People's Daily*, May 1, 2020.

Index

Printed and bound by CPI Group (UK) Ltd, Croydon, CR0 4YY

14/11/2023

08188986-0001